Suzannah Olivier

ALLERGY

SOLUTIONS

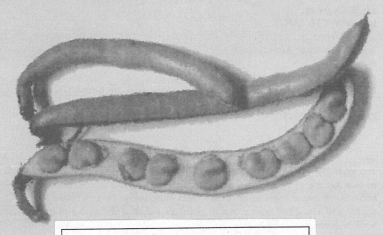

POCKET
B O O K S

First published in Great Britain by Pocket Books, 2001
An imprint of Simon & Schuster UK Ltd
A Viacom Company

10 9 8 7 6 5 4 3 2 1

Simon & Schuster UK Ltd
Africa House
64-78 Kingsway
London WC2B 6AH

Simon & Schuster Australia
Sydney

A CIP catalogue record for this book is available from the British Library

ISBN 0-671-77313-5

You must always consult your doctor for an accurate diagnosis of an allergy,
to rule out any more serious conditions, before using the information in this
book. Significant changes to children's diets must always be supervised by a
doctor and a qualified nutritionist or dietician. None of the advice in this
book is suitable for pregnant or breastfeeding women.

Typeset in 12 on 14pt Perpetua with Gill Sans display
Design and page make-up by Peter Ward
Printed and bound in Great Britain by Omnia Books Limited, Glasgow

For *the* Laurence Olivier

Contents

Part One

ALLERGY FACTS

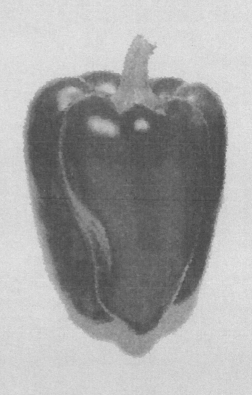

CHAPTER ONE

The Allergy Epidemic

Each year the number of people with allergies continues to rise – nobody is quite sure why, though there are several theories. No two health disciplines seem to agree on how to treat them though, again, there are many views. It seems likely that there are a number of effective ways of treating allergies and that different treatments may be suited to different people. Underscoring this is the fact that making dietary changes is likely to be a successful part of the treatment for many allergy sufferers. I have certainly seen profound improvements in the health of people who have been struggling with allergies for many years and who have been told that it is just something they have to live with, or that they might eventually grow out of. This example is fairly typical: one four-year-old boy with asthma, who was using his inhaler several times a week, had an identified allergy to house dust mites. When his parents made significant changes to his diet, they were able to reduce the use of his inhaler to a couple of times a month. In some people, dietary changes can directly influence allergy symptoms and result in reasonably prompt and complete relief, often within a few weeks. In others, while total relief is elusive because of the nature of their allergy, significant improvement in the management of their symptoms is possible. In addition, they experience an improvement in their general state of health.

Allergies can be life-threatening and for some are a serious daily worry. Even milder allergies can be debilitating and restrictive, and the source of many problems. Our very survival depends on a constant war being waged between ourselves and the outside world, and it is our immune system which is responsible for protecting us from any assault from the outside. The allergy reaction is one facet of the working of the immune system, and is a result of the outside world successfully encroaching, to one degree or another, on our inside world. Every second that we are on this earth we are threatened by invaders – bacteria, yeast, viruses, parasites, poisons and pollutants – and every second our bodies must repel these potential invaders to maintain our equilibrium.

As the statistics for allergies are soaring it seems that things are going badly in this hidden war. Why are allergies dramatically on the increase? Worsening air pollution and modern stress levels undoubtedly contribute, as do the increasing number of chemicals with which we come into daily contact. Allergies are, by and large, diseases of an affluent society. If you live in a well-off Western country, particularly in a large city, your chances of having an allergy are very high.

Here are some disturbing facts:

- Over 40 per cent of the population suffer from allergies.
- In the last 20 years, asthma cases have soared from 3 per cent of the population to 10 per cent.
- During the same time, the number of people suffering from hay fever has risen from 6 per cent to 20 per cent of the population.
- Eczema affects one in eight children and one in ten of the general population.
- At a conservative estimate, one in 200 children has a peanut allergy.
- Four out of ten children under the age of six suffer with glue ear (otitis media).
- Acute severe allergy probably affects 1–2 per cent of the UK population (500,000–1 million people) and one in

6,000 casualty cases involves anaphylaxis (a severe immune reaction).

These alarming statistics are the reality with which we must now deal. Apart from the massive increases in asthma, hay fever, eczema and other conditions, allergies to foods such as peanuts and shellfish are becoming more common, with severe and, in a few cases, fatal results. A tiny minority of people, are even said to suffer 'total allergy syndrome' or 'multiple chemical sensitivity', and react to an overwhelming number of man-made substances, including latex, adhesives and metals. It seems we could be in danger of becoming aliens on our own planet.

Of course, there is the possibility that there has been an over-diagnosis of allergies. If nothing else seems to be wrong, the condition is often blamed on an allergy. Certainly some natural health practitioners can be guilty of doing this, as can the medical profession, perhaps in part due to limited consultation times available within the health service in the UK. I certainly had a nasty moment when my son was diagnosed as a possible asthmatic, when all he had was a recurrent upper respiratory tract infection. If I had accepted the proffered medication we might be on the road to a suppressed immune system from the side-effects of the steroid drugs on offer. In the months after this near-miss diagnosis I spoke to no less than six parents who had had the same experience and who, mostly, had put their children on six months of needless, and ineffective, medication.

Of course, drugs can be lifesavers and, at the very least, tremendously soothing. To a person in the throws of an anaphylactic reaction, involving swelling of the air tubes, an adrenaline injection can mean the difference between life and death. An inhaler loaded with corticosteroids can stop a severe asthma attack in its tracks. If a child with eczema is scratching herself to the point where she bleeds, cortisone cream can diminish the inflammation and itching to tolerable levels, enough to ensure an uninterrupted night's sleep. But none of these will get rid of the allergy and allow the person to avoid being counted as one of the statistics. More needs to be done to uncover the underlying contributors to the condition and, for many people, finding the nutritional factors that are contributing to the allergy is the only long-term, truly effective route that will make the difference.

CHAPTER TWO

What Are Allergies?

Allergies are 'altered' immune reactions. When your immune system reacts adversely to a substance that does not normally create a reaction in most people, this is an allergy.

Classic allergies involve immune reactions that have been 'programmed'. When an allergic person is exposed to an allergen (allergy-causing substance) the immune system of that person is programmed to react when re-exposed to it. The severity of symptoms depends upon how strong this reaction is.

Our first lines of defence against the outside world are our skin, the lining of our digestive tract, and the mucus membranes that line our airways, mouth, ears, eye sockets, urinary tract, anus and vagina. These create a continuous physical barrier to keep foreign substances at bay. In susceptible people, allergic reactions happen:

● when the surface membranes are unusually sensitive to certain chemicals or foreign substances that other people can usually tolerate, such as pollen, house dust mites and animal hair and skin (dander), with resultant irritation and inflammation of the area;
● or when the barrier is breached – for example when an insect sting penetrates the skin or when a particular food protein molecule crosses the digestive barrier into the bloodstream.

Our bodies are constantly keeping checks and maintaining balances, dealing with the numerous assaults that happen. For the most part, the body's defence mechanisms do not allow an immune reaction to get out of hand in a way that would lead to serious damage. But when it does get out of control, life-threatening situations can result, as in the case of an anaphylactic reaction where the airways close up from swelling that has resulted from, for example, exposure to peanuts. Another way in which the immune system can get out of control occurs in auto-immune diseases, such as rheumatoid arthritis, where the immune system begins to attack joint tissues causing inflammation and joint problems.

ATOPIC FAMILIES

A tendency to allergic reactions can run in families – in other words there can be a genetic predisposition to being a sufferer. This is called atopy, and families who are genetically prone to allergies are referred to as atopic families. If both parents have a history of atopy, the chances of a child being affected is 50 per cent; if one parent is atopic, there is a 30 per cent chance of a child having atopic allergies; but if neither parent is affected there is still a 10–12 per cent chance of a child having allergy problems.

But there the logic of atopic families ends, and a number of different types of allergies can come to the fore with different family members. One person may have asthma, another hay fever, yet another urticaria (nettle rash), or eczema, or a food allergy, and so on. Atopic allergies can skip generations, and to look for clues you may need to work out if your aunts, uncles, cousins or grandparents were atopic, as your parents may not exhibit any signs.

Just as confusingly, it is common for allergies to change in one person. For instance, a child may have an allergy to milk or atopic eczema, and then grow out of it. But in later years the same person will often develop a new allergy such as asthma, hay fever or allergic colitis. It is as if their body has overcome the first allergy and managed to maintain the status quo for a while, only to be overwhelmed again at a later date. They seem to manage in the face of regular exposure to foods or substances to which they are sensitive, but only up to a point.

THE PROBLEMS OF OVERLOAD

While a genetic tendency is an important factor in the causation of allergy, there are other factors to consider in the nutritional treatment of allergy. An important principle to understand is that of overload. Genetics may play a part, but that is not all there is to it. The increase we have seen in recent years in the number of asthmatics and hay fever sufferers points firmly to other influences playing a major part.

The immune system can cope up to a point, but if too much is expected of it, because it has either been overwhelmed or because it has not been given the raw materials it needs to do its job, it begins to malfunction and either becomes suppressed or overreacts. This in part explains the situation described above, whereby a childhood allergy disappears only to reappear later in another form. The body has learned to cope, but as the person ages and overloads their system with, for instance, too many late nights, an irregular diet, stress at work, alcohol, smoking or overuse of antibiotics, the body eventually reacts again. This is discussed in greater detail in **Supporting Your Immune System**, page 45.

The accumulation of factors that weaken the body's defence systems, such as mental and emotional stresses, dietary deficiencies and excessive physical demands, impact on the working of the body's stress management system – the adrenal glands and the hormones produced by them, adrenaline and cortisol.

I shall review the importance of this later in **The Stress Factor**, page 25.

THE ALLERGY REACTION

The immune system is our defence mechanism against harm from foreign substances. It can be thought of as an army which is constantly patrolling the territory in order to identify, mark, destroy and despatch invaders. The immune system reacts to:

- particles to which we may be sensitive (eg pollen);
- chemicals to which we may be sensitive (eg in washing powder);
- incompletely digested food particles that may cross the gut wall;
- bacteria, viruses and parasites to which we are exposed;
- dead cells that have outlived their usefulness;
- cancer cells which have mutated and must be destroyed before they can grow out of control.

In order for the immune system to decide whether it needs to set in train defensive measures, it must first identify the 'invader' – in other words distinguish between friend and foe. It generally does this by recognising the arrangement of proteins, or particular chemicals, on an antigen's surface. An antigen is simply a molecule that stimulates the immune system to react. For example, the markers on the surface of a dangerous salmonella bacterium will be quite different to those of friendly lactobacilli bacteria that colonise our gut walls and upon which we depend for a number of health-giving properties. The salmonella must be identified and destroyed, while the beneficial bacteria must be allowed to establish themselves and thrive. If the antigen contains proteins that stimulate an allergic reaction, then the antigen is called an allergen. An allergen is simply an antigen which stimulates an allergic reaction.

The immune system is made up of a number of components:

- the bone marrow and thymus where white blood cells are made and programmed for their specific immune functions;
- the lymph system and blood system, in which the white blood cells patrol and get to their destinations;
- the lymph glands, which trap 'foes' to be despatched by white blood cells;
- the gut wall, which contains large amounts of lymph tissue and produces immune compounds;
- 120 million white blood cells, which identify, tag, destroy and clear up invaders such as bacteria, viruses, dead cells and mutated cells (about one million white blood cells are produced each minute when an immune defence is mounted);
- and various antioxidant enzymes produced in the body which protect our cells from general oxidation damage, including the damage that occurs when allergic inflammation sets in.

Ensuring the health of all of these components of the immune system is an important factor in the successful treatment of allergies (see **Supporting Your Immune System**, page 45).

TRIGGER HAPPY

When an allergen triggers an immune response, the immune system produces specialised proteins called antibodies. Each type of antibody is programmed to launch an attack on one specific allergen only, for example grass pollen. However, in some cases, a substance can be sufficiently similar to another to be able to fool the immune system into triggering an immune reaction. For example, the true allergy may be to grass pollen, causing hay fever, but other grasses, such as wheat or rye in the diet, may make the hay fever sufferer more sensitive.

Also involved in our immune defence reactions are several different classes of immunoglobulins. Immunoglobulins are called Ig for short – IgM, IgA, IgD, IgG, IgE – hence the acronym MADGE. They all have different functions, but for our purposes the IgE reaction is the most important as it is involved in what are known as classic allergic reactions. IgE is a bit of a troublemaker, as it has a strong affinity with some specialised cells in the body, called mast cells and basophils.

Mast cells lie along blood vessels and are found primarily in the skin, in the airways of the lungs and in the gastrointestinal tract. These cells produce irritating and damaging chemicals, including histamine.

IgE stimulates the release of these chemicals, which the body uses to get rid of offending substances – for instance to flush out pollen from the nasal passages. This process causes the blood vessels to dilate, which in turn causes the nose lining to become red and inflamed, and for mucus production to be stepped up. This leads to the blocked noses, watering eyes, sneezing and itchy throats that are typical symptoms of hay fever.

Histamine is involved in many allergic reactions where there is reddening, irritation and inflammation. While IgE molecules are the main triggers of mast cells they are not the only ones, and different triggers may account for different levels of allergic reactions. Basophils are types of white blood cells which move around in the blood (as opposed to being fixed like mast cells) and which also contain histamine and are triggered in allergy reactions.

Histamine can be found in a number of foods and hypersensitive people may find that they react to histamine in foods as well (see **Reducing Your Histamine Reaction**, page 63, and **Appendices**, page 171). It is also found in stinging nettles, and the red, itchy bump that a nettle sting can cause gives an idea of its effect and potency.

Histamine has another function, however: that of a nerve transmitter or 'messenger' between brain cells. Drugs that block the action of histamine to relieve allergy problems can cause drowsiness, because by blocking histamine release by the mast cells they simultaneously block the action of histamine in the brain.

INFLAMED PASSIONS

The process of inflammation is natural, and it should also be beneficial. Inflammation occurs, principally, as a natural reaction to protect an area, and the pain it causes is a warning to avoid creating further damage. If you cut yourself, the inflammation acts as a sort of natural bandage to the area telling you to take care. It also increases the blood supply to the area, providing nutrients for healing. Inflammation also has an important preventive effect by keeping foreign matter from leaving the site of the trouble and spreading around the body. Problems occur when a person finds themselves in a hyper-inflammatory state as a result of the inflammation mechanism getting out of control. The most obvious example of this is in rheumatoid arthritis, but you see it also when wounds and ulcers fail to heal quickly and effectively. Since inflammation is a major symptom of allergy and sensitivity, this situation can also arise in people with allergies.

The important message to remember is that it is all a question of balance. Our bodies produce chemicals that are geared to regulate inflammation. If the balance between these chemicals is correct, inflammation takes place in an appropriate way.

The main chemicals involved in controlling the inflammation process are prostaglandins and leukotrienes. For now, all that we need to understand is that some of these chemicals promote inflammation, while others dampen it down. The other important fact to understand is that fats in the diet *directly influence* the balance of these chemicals. This is one of the better understood mechanisms of dietary manipulation, and one which helps us to make very specific recommendations about how to reduce the inflammation that is typical of allergic reactions. For a full run down on how to influence the production of beneficial prostaglandins and suppress unhelpful prostaglandins and leukotrienes see **Understanding Fats**, page 52.

CHAPTER THREE

When Is An Allergy Not An Allergy?

Classical allergy reactions, as already discussed, involve an IgE immune reaction. If this was all there was to allergies, life would be relatively simple, but unfortunately that is not the case. A whole spectrum of reactions – some of which involve a different type of immune reaction and others which do not – are implicated in 'allergic' health problems. It is estimated that classic IgE food allergies only occur in about 1.5 per cent of the population, and that other adverse food reactions are caused by food sensitivities or intolerances.

One type of food reaction, which does not involve the immune system, occurs where there is an enzyme deficiency, meaning that a particular food cannot be metabolised. About 10–15 per cent of the population of northern and middle Europe have a deficiency in the milk sugar enzyme, lactase, which can lead to uncomfortable bloating whenever milk and high lactose milk-based foods are eaten. Amongst southern European, Asian, Hispanic, Jewish and African-descent populations as many as 65–95 per cent have the enzyme missing or much reduced. Another common enzyme deficiency results in certain foods high in compounds called amines triggering migraines.

Beyond a few agreed definitions of allergy and intolerance, there is little agreement amongst the medical profession about other types of reactions to food sensitivities and intolerances. Yet many people are coming forward with health problems that are resolved by avoiding certain foods, and sufficient cases have now been observed by doctors and allergy experts for them to be taken seriously. But because tests do not definitively explain the response to the food or foods, the reactions are called 'idiopathic', which simply means without explanation. At least they are being acknowledged, whereas at one time these people would have been dismissed with 'it's all in your mind'. Of course, there are cases of psychologically-based food aversions and some placebo effects to improving diet, but for the majority of cases it is a demonstrable fact that certain foods cause specific or generalised adverse reactions in certain people, which clear up when the foods are avoided and are replicated when reintroduced. As far as the person who is experiencing these adverse food reactions is concerned they are merely allergic reactions by another name.

'True' allergy and food intolerance or sensitivity have different patterns of adverse responses. The following is a summary of the likely differences:

Classical or fixed reaction allergy	Delayed sensitivity or intolerance
a small number of foods (typically one or two) trigger the reaction	not unusual for a few types of foods to be involved
usually involves infrequently eaten foods	usually involves foods most commonly eaten
allergic symptoms usually appear within 2 hours of exposure to the offending food	reactions can appear anything up to 72 hours after consumption

Classical or fixed reaction allergy	Delayed sensitivity or intolerance
primarily affects the digestive tract, airways and skin	almost any system may be affected and reactions can include seemingly unrelated symptoms
usually does not involve addiction to the foods or withdrawal symptoms	often involves addiction to the offending foods and withdrawal symptoms
tiny amounts of the food can trigger a significant, and sometimes serious, reaction	reactions usually triggered by eating larger amounts of the foods or by eating them regularly
often the allergy remains fixed, or permanent	adverse reactions can often be eliminated by avoiding the foods for 2–6 months, and sensitivity may be reversed totally with careful management
often tests positive on skin prick tests, IgE ELISA/RAST blood tests (see Allergy Tests, page 178).	usually test negative to skin prick, IgE ELISA/RAST tests, but can test positive to IgG ELISA/RAST tests (see Allergy Tests, page 178).

IgG is the most abundant antibody in the body and deals with antibody production against micro-organisms such as bacteria and viruses, but it is also involved in food sensitivities. An IgG immune reaction to food is quite different to an IgE allergic reaction, but may be just as troublesome. The reaction is usually delayed, which makes it all the more difficult to track down. Working out what may be causing the symptoms you are experiencing is not easy if the reactions occur several hours, or even a couple of days, after eating the food. Sometimes it can involve the most unlikely foods, as well as the most commonly eaten ones. This sort of reaction to foods can undermine health in the most surreptitious way, affecting any number of body 'systems', such as the digestive system, the immune system, the respiratory system, the nervous system, and so on.

An IgG reaction is a type of immune response that has only a short-term memory. A food can trigger an IgG response, but if the food is avoided for 6–8 weeks, the IgG response is usually 'forgotten' by the immune system. The IgG response is not then reprogrammed unless the food is eaten regularly for several consecutive days. The food can, theoretically, be reintroduced and, as long as it is not eaten more than one day in four or five, will not reprogramme a reaction. While the IgG reaction is often life-long, it can be controlled in the short term by this means.

Possible symptoms of food intolerances and sensitivities

acne	headaches
addictions	heartburn
arthritis (esp RA)	hives
asthma	hot flushes
belching or gas	hyperactivity
bloated feeling	insomnia

breast pain	joint aches
congestion	migraines
constipation	muscle pain
cravings	mood swings
depression	nausea
diarrhoea	PMS/PMT
dry or watery eyes	rapid heartbeat
ear infections	sinusitis
eczema	stomach cramp
eye circles	sweating
fatigue	tinnitus
genital itch	water retention
hay fever	weight gain

One man who, it is reported, is currently being considered for an entry in the *Guinness Book of Records* is believed to have sneezed more or less continuously for 37 years, making his life miserable and, in his words, exhausting. He had all the standard allergy tests, which came up with nothing, and was prescribed steroid drugs which resulted in thinned bones (osteoporosis). He finally had a non-orthodox test for IgG and discovered that he was sensitive (amongst other foods) to the oats in his morning muesli. As soon as he gave up eating these foods his 37-year sneezing fit stopped, meaning he could at last sleep properly and relax. An IgG blood test is often inconclusive, but it can, as in this case, lead to a correct diagnosis and successful result (see **Allergy Tests**, page 178). And while this is a particularly extreme case, identifying food intolerances can play a major part in the treatment of many people with allergies.

Even those who also have classical IgE reactions can benefit from identifying IgG food reactions, since an IgG reaction can have the effect of aggravating an IgE 'true' allergy reaction, as in the case of cereal foods which often intensify hay fever symptoms. Part of the problem is that the intolerances can undermine the immune system and sufficiently damage health to make the IgE reaction worse. If you manage to eliminate the IgG problem the IgE reaction is often significantly reduced.

Whether an allergy is a 'true' allergy or an 'idiopathic' one (more accurately referred to as a sensitivity), just about any food is capable of triggering an unpleasant physical reaction. The best known allergen is the peanut; other common ones are nuts of all sorts, grains (particularly wheat), soya, sesame, eggs, milk, oranges, fish and shellfish. Virtuallly any food can act as an allergen, however, even those we think of as innocuous – examples I have come across include camomile tea (a relative of ragweed) and bean sprouts.

It can be difficult to find out what foods may be triggering your symptoms. It is not unheard of to react to a food in its raw state, but not the cooked version, or to find that two events must take place to elicit a reaction, for example eating the food, and then exercising. It may not be the food that is causing the problem – the reaction could be to traces of latex from rubber gloves used by food handlers, or to some other contaminant or parasite (particularly in fish or shellfish) or to a food additive.

If you are sensitive to a known food, one of the possibilities to look out for is that you may also react to other foods in the same family. It is not always obvious which foods belong to the same families so, if in doubt, refer to **Appendices**, page 164, which details the food families of the most frequently eaten foods. On the other hand, it is also very common to be sensitive to one food, and yet be able to eat other foods from the same family. It is really a matter of trial and error to find out into which category you fit.

HIDDEN ALLERGY

Clinical ecologists, who are doctors with an interest in how the environment can make us ill or well (and this includes the foods we eat), have championed the theory of hidden allergies for years – to the derision of conventional allergists, who do not recognise this phenomenon.

The term hidden allergy refers to a substance to which a person is sufficiently allergic or sensitive for it to be capable of making them ill, though constant exposure to the substance may render the negative reaction less severe. The person might then feel under par, but not definitely ill. Avoiding the substance relieves related health problems, but if this is followed by fresh exposure a more dramatic reaction can occur. Alternatively, if the person is still exposed to the substance, other taxing circumstances, such as stress, illness or pollution can trigger more serious sensitivity to the substance which is responsible for the hidden allergy.

It was Dr Herbert Rinkel, an allergist and one of the fathers of the clinical ecology approach, who first observed this series of events in relation to his own health. As a mature medical student, he suffered badly with catarrh. Like many students, he was broke, and his father sent him crates of eggs from the family farm in Kansas. Throughout his studies he never felt totally well. He suspected the eggs but his impoverished condition meant that he carried on eating them. Years later, Rinkel noticed that if he ate many eggs at once he felt really unwell. At one point he avoided eggs totally and found that, for the first time, he felt much better. A few days later he ate some cake made with eggs, and fell unconscious having to be revived with an adrenalin shot. He realised that while he had been eating eggs for many years the allergy had been 'masked', only for it to appear in full force from a small exposure after avoiding them for some time.

This is actually a very common phenomenon. Someone who

avoids a food for a period of time, and finds it relieves their symptoms, can have a particularly unpleasant reaction to it when it is reintroduced. This is the complete reverse of the situation, described previously, whereby a food can be tolerated, in reduced quantities and in rotation, after it has been avoided for a while. Which reaction you are likely to have can only be ascertained by avoiding the food and then reintroducing it. The one thing that is certain is that if you correctly identify foods that are implicated in your ill health, avoiding them can make you feel a lot better, with partial or complete remission of symptoms.

Part Two

OTHER FACTORS

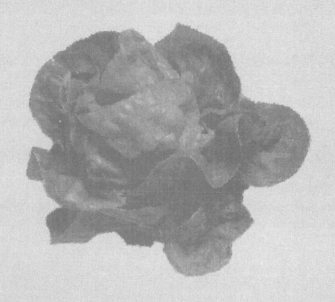

CHAPTER FOUR

The Stress Factor

Stress has become the watchword of our time. As with all fashionable ailments, however, there is always scepticism, and inevitably some people question the importance of stress in relation to allergies – after all the human race has been subjected to it for eons. But the nature of stress has undoubtedly changed. Whereas once our stress reaction was primed to deal with the need to gather food, find shelter and warmth, and protect ourselves from predators, now it is common to experience constant low-to-moderate stress throughout the day, the effects of which can accumulate. The commuter rush, anxieties at work, pressure on time and finances, and the constant need to make decisions in the face of a bombardment of information can grind us down. It is even possile to get addicted to this level of stress, hence our attempts to unwind by reading thriller novels and taking adventure holidays.

Stress is intimately linked to allergic reactions. The adrenal glands, which produce our stress hormones, also produce the anti-inflammatory cortisone steroid hormones which are needed to balance these. To counteract allergic reactions your doctor may well prescribe some of these steroid hormones, such as in inhalers for asthma, or cortisone cream for eczema. If an acute anaphylactic shock reaction is taking place, it is the life-saving compound adrenaline, the stress hormone made by the adrenal glands, that is injected. So it is easy to see that the health of the adrenal glands, which produce these hormones, is of prime importance in treating allergies naturally.

In the 1930s Hans Selyé, the 'grandfather of stress',

conducted experiments on rats to investigate their hormone reactions – though the hormone he was actually intending to find out about was oestrogen. (In fact, an astoundingly high number of scientific and drug discoveries have been made by observing events which have occurred as a part of experiments in quite different fields – Viagra, for instance, was originally investigated as a potential heart medication.) As the story goes, Selyé, who was on the clumsy side, had the unfortunate habit of dropping these hapless rats and having to fish them out from behind the filing cabinets with a broom. Not surprisingly, these rats were stressed. Selyé noticed that the adrenal glands of the rats he was studying had grown large – a condition known as hypertrophy. He discovered that in response to chronic stress the adrenal glands enlarge and try to push out more and more adrenal hormones to compensate. If this carries on for too long, the adrenal glands become 'functionally depleted', and are unable to maintain this high level of output. The reverse then happens and the level of adrenal hormones drops. A consequence of this is that the allergic inflammatory reaction is less easily dampened down.

The degree to which this happens varies enormously from person to person, and some people are able to take greater amounts of stress than others. It is quite likely that those who suffer from allergic reactions have less ability to cope physically with the onslaught of stress – in other words they are unable to maintain their levels of hormones – and that part of their adverse reaction to stress is exhibited in allergic reactions. One of the most important steps to take when combating allergies is to nurture your adrenal glands, with the aim of improving their output of steroid hormones (see **Supporting Your Adrenal Function**, page 62).

Remember, also, the effects of stress on children in relation to their allergies. I have seen countless children with severe eczema and asthma whose parents are understandably anxious and who have sought to remedy their children's condition with a nutritional approach. It sometimes becomes clear, in the course of the consultation, that either the parents are of an anxious disposition and that great pressure is being brought to bear on the child, or that there is discord at home (often about the treatment strategy) and that this is having an adverse effect on the child's anxiety and stress levels. In such circumstances, nutritional treatment can have only limited effect, and it is necessary to encourage the family to alter their behavioural patterns.

Chronic stress has a negative impact on the immune system, and it is the immune system that needs to be kept healthy to reduce the impact of allergies. Adrenaline is our emergency hormone, designed to prepare our bodies to protect ourselves from danger. Because of this life-saving function, the production of stress hormones takes priority over many other functions in the body. Producing adrenaline is also quite an 'expensive' task, using up lots of the nutrients that might otherwise be used by the immune system – nutrients such as the B-complex vitamins and vitamin C, and minerals such as zinc and magnesium. By robbing the immune system of these nutrients, overall health is impaired, and we can become more vulnerable to the onslaught of 'foreign bodies', and thus the likelihood of allergic-type reactions increases.

Nutritional measures to support your immune system are discussed in **Strategies For Allergies**, page 39. For the moment, however, it is worth thinking about what you can do to reduce the stress in your life. Never underestimate the advantages of cutting back on chronic stress and learning how you can relax as often as possible as a means of managing allergy problems.

STEROID MEDICATION

One of the main classes of drugs used for the management of allergies is steroids. These mimic our natural steroid hormones, but are a bit of a chemical cosh. One of the problems of using steroid medication for asthma, and to a lesser degree in creams for eczema, is that prolonged usage, or high doses, are likely to lead to adrenal suppression. The adrenal glands give up working as effectively as they ought to, and they do not regain their capability when the long-term medication is withdrawn. For this reason some patients who have had long-term steroid medication may be given emergency cards to carry with them so that they can receive steroid drugs if they are under stress, for example during an operation, when their adrenal sufficiency may not be enough to carry them through such a procedure.

Obviously steroids may be needed at times of crisis, however the responsible approach must be to find the underlying cause of the problem in order to prevent long-term damage from strong medication. Supporting adrenal health is of paramount importance when attempting to achieve an allergy-free life or a reduction in the severity of reactions (see **Supporting Your Adrenal Function**, page 62).

REDUCING STRESS IN YOUR LIFE

You've heard it all before – you need to get rid of some of the stress in your life and learn to relax more. But have you done it? What is stopping you? This is a book about nutrition and allergies, and really the subject of stress and allergies merits a whole book in its own right! All I aim to do here is to give you a checklist of the factors to consider within the context of your own life. Work on only one of the aspects at a time, perhaps one a week, or even one a month. For more guidance on stress management see **Resources** at the end of this book.

- If you are plagued by emotional worries, find someone to confide in. While a friendly ear can be sufficient, you may need to find someone who is able to help you work out the best way forward.
- Learn to relax. *Really* learn to relax. This is a habit just as much as any other. Make time for yourself daily (just 15 minutes twice a day will help) and be selfish about it. If you can't get any peace at home or at the office, go out and find somewhere where you can (the library, a park bench, a café). Don't do anything with that time other than meditate. We often fill every gap of time with just one more job, but allow yourself the time to refresh and you will be twice as effective at other times.
- Finding time for ourselves is one of the hardest things to do, but also the most valuable. If you find yourself saying 'but I still have to deal with the kids' or 'I need to look after my ageing parent' you need to find a means by which you can absolve yourself of some of that responsibility for a short period each day – swap with a friend, or find a new friend you can swap with through a self-help group of people with the same interests/problems.
- There is nothing quite so beneficial as fresh air, sunlight and rest to your overall health.
- Take holidays. If you can't afford to go away, take a holiday at home. Take the phone off the hook, cancel the papers with all their stressful news, unplug the TV and give yourself a project that will distract you from your problems – paint a picture, paint a room, do the crossword, tidy your wardrobe, give yourself a beauty salon treatment. Anything that is different from your daily routine and which will make you feel good.
- Illness is disharmony. Always seek ways to restore harmony. Melody and rhythm are powerful ways to restore

harmony. Sing in the shower, listen to music, attend a concert or conduct an orchestra in your mind. If there is discord or disharmony in your life, with your partner or due to financial or work worries, you will need to work on it from a practical point of view, but in the meantime use music, art therapy or gentle movement such as yoga or tai chi, to give some balance and harmony to your life.

CHAPTER FIVE

The Pollution Factor

As humans, we need three basic ingredients to thrive – clean water, clean food and clean air. The last of these three is hard to guarantee these days, and it can sometimes seem as if we are suffocating ourselves. The quality of the air we breathe is bound to have an effect on our overall health, and this includes allergy reactions, because we need a good clean oxygen supply simply to function. If we live in a polluted inner city or an area of frequent crop spraying this inevitably impacts on our health.

It is obvious to most people that pollution must be involved in the problems of asthma and hay fever, as attacks rocket on days when pollution is at its worse, but how can pollution have any bearing on other allergies? It depends on what you call pollution. The type of pollution that is normally referred to is caused by car and factory emissions. But of course we pollute our world in many other ways. Our exposure to pollution is actually much worse within our homes, which are hermetically sealed against heat loss, and therefore also against the dispersion of chemicals, so levels build up dramatically. This sort of pollution, in addition to the air-quality pollution, and the thousands of chemicals we come into contact with in our food and water, has an impact on other allergy problems. Once again it is the problem of overload.

Even personal products, which you might think of as innocuous, can be a hazard. Many allergic people are hypersensitive to perfumes, and this includes those in shampoos, body washes, after-shaves, bath products and washing powders. Again, the closed environment of our homes means that the chemicals found in these products recirculates and contributes further to the problem. Even so-called hypoallergenic formulas can harbour chemicals and perfumes to which you may be sensitive. There are, however, several truly chemical- and perfume-free products now available (see **Resources**, page 188).

In addition, many people have wall-to-wall carpeting, something that is very popular with the house dust mite. Apart from being involved in asthma, house dust mite allergy is also linked to rhinitis, as well as to the majority of eczema cases. For measures that can help to keep the house dust mite at bay see below.

GRUBBY MAY BE GOOD

There is another good reason to abandon the many sprays and fluids with which we clean our homes. One of the theories as to why there has been such an increase in the rates of asthma and hay fever in westernised countries is that we have become too sanitised. Our homes are too clean, we are exposed to far less dirt and fewer germs as children, and consequently do not go through the necessary early priming of the immune system. Subsequently, our bodies overreact to things that should be harmless, such as dust, pollen and foods. To quote one newspaper article, 'It is as if the human immune system, deprived of a decent infection or two to fight in the modern, sterile world, is turning in on itself for a bit of self-destructive mayhem.'

Many people feel nervous at the thought of abandoning chemical disinfectants and deodorisers, and advertisers contribute to the worry we feel about the cleanliness of our homes and the germs lurking in them. Yet it is these very germs that might be useful in priming our immune systems when we are young. In general, it is best to keep cleaning routines thorough but simple. What was once achieved by soap and a scrubbing brush now takes several different anti-bacterial sprays. Instead, try using simply water and washing up liquid, borax, white wine vinegar (good for getting rid of moulds) and some tea tree oil or grapefruit seed extract (see **Resources**, page 185, for further information).

ASTHMA AND POLLUTION

It is generally believed that pollution is intimately linked to asthma, but this is not necessarily the case. Both the UK and New Zealand appear at the top of the league of countries with asthma sufferers. While both countries share similar Western diets, there is an interesting, and crucial, difference between the two. Air pollution rates in the UK are high, but in New Zealand they are negligible. Outdoor pollution may therefore have less to do with asthma than we thought after all. On the other hand, we share indoor pollution levels with other industrialised countries. One paper noted that urban residents can spend 20–22 hours per day indoors, during which time they are exposed to dust, mites and household chemicals. Perhaps we just need to get out more. Certainly asthma remains rare in countries where outdoor life is the norm. Recent research has also made a strong link between diet and asthma, so perhaps we are now seeing confirmation that diet is more critical, or at least as critical, a cause of asthma as other factors. This does not deny the importance of reducing pollution levels, but supports the importance of diet.

There are many airborne triggers for asthma apart from pollution, and these are some of the most important to keep a check on:

Smoking
Stop smoking and avoid smoky atmospheres. If you are one of the one in four women who continue to smoke during pregnancy

please stop, as there is an increased risk of asthma in your child if you continue.

Dust

Reduce your exposure to dust, as it contains various potential allergens, the main one being the house dust mite and its faeces. If your mattress is old, replace it. Buy non-allergenic duvet, pillows and covers. Ideally replace any carpets with hard flooring (wood or tile), because wall-to-wall carpeting means wall-to-wall dust mites. If you cannot do this, vacuum the carpet at least twice weekly, with a special vacuum cleaner designed for allergy sufferers. Most vacuum cleaners have been shown to blow 60–70 per cent of the dust back into the atmosphere, so it is well worth investing in a vacuum specially designed for allergy sufferers (see **Resources**, page 188). Damp dust all surfaces at least once a week. The tannin in tea combines, chemically, with the house dust mite faeces, reducing their allergic potential to asthmatics. Spray a fine mist of strong tea (no milk!) on surfaces and mattresses that collect dust. Clothing and bedding can be washed in your machine using a eucalyptus mixture which has been shown to kill 97–99 per cent of mites. Make a solution with 4 parts eucalyptus oil and emulsify with 1 part dishwashing liquid. The study used a 0.2 per cent solution (with washing powder) in the machine for 30–60 minutes – in practice you may find it hard to measure this out precisely so you may have to use trial and error. Another option is to do a very hot wash at 60° C using a few of drops of tea tree oil.

Make your bedroom a dust and mite free zone

You spend one-third of your life in your bedroom, so it stands to reason that this is the most important area to clean up.

Vacuum your mattress once or twice weekly, and cover it with a close fitting anti-allergenic cover. Avoid putting soft, cuddly toys in the bed with asthmatic children. Clean away any areas to which dust is attracted – get rid of pelmets, curtains, lightshades, books and clutter on shelves, put doors on wardrobes and have a simple wooden headboard. Vacuum in all corners, crevices and under the bed at least once a week. Avoid fan heaters, convection and open bar heaters, all of which recirculate dust. Anti-mite paints might be effective for woodwork, but since 99 per cent of mites live in fabrics the overall effect is likely to be minimal. Heating encourages mites to breed, so keep your bedroom cooler than other rooms.

Animal fur and feathers
Avoid contact with animals or animal hair that may trigger an attack. Cat dander (hair and skin) causes more problems than dog dander, and contact with other animals, including horses, can also lead to attacks.

Grasses and pollens
Not only can these lead to hay fever, but they can also be implicated in asthma. Pollen counts are higher on warm and dry days. When the pollen count warnings are high it may be best to stay indoors. On the other hand, being by the seaside can make the situation much better. Ionizers, which produce negatively-charged ions (such as those found by the sea), and which cause dust to settle instead of staying in the air, may help a little, though they are not to be relied upon as the sole means of reducing dust.

Moulds
If you are sensitive to moulds, it is important to check to see if your house has any patches – sensitive areas include bathrooms,

cellars, kitchens, basement areas and ground floor rooms where there may be rising damp. Mildew and damp areas need to be appropriately treated.

Chemicals

These can also trigger asthma, although they are a less common cause. If you suspect it may be a problem, clear out all chemicals, sprays, washing powders, paints, photocopiers, etc, from your house, garden and work place to ascertain if this makes a difference. You could use a product for years and then suddenly become hypersensitive to it, so do not assume that if you have used a product for ages, and have been fine in the past, that this is still the case. Keep a draught going through your home, with windows open at both ends of the building, for at least a few hours a day, to prevent chemical fumes from building up in your home. This will also disperse fumes if you regularly burn fires. On high pollen or pollution days, or if you are very vulnerable to temperature changes, you may not be able to do this quite so often, but it is generally still a good discipline, and at least you should be able to open the windows at night without any problems.

Part Three

STRATEGIES

FOR ALLERGIES

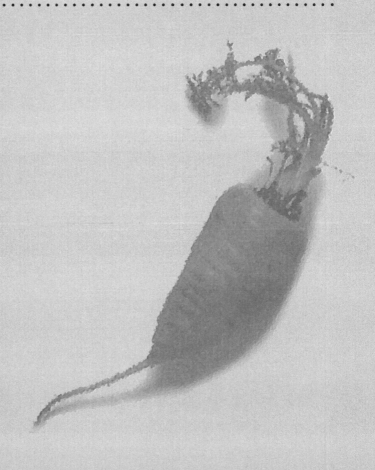

CHAPTER SIX

Strategies For Allergies

There are several common factors that underlie the allergic condition which means, from a nutritional standpoint, that there are common factors that can be addressed with the diet. In this chapter we will look at the five most important of these:

- Avoiding foods that compound the allergy
- Supporting your immune system
- Nutrients needed for skin and mucus membrane health
- Reducing inflammation
- Reducing histamine levels

While the terms 'allergy', 'intolerance' and 'sensitivity' all mean different things, for the sake of ease, and so as not to involve too much repetition, I will mainly use the umbrella term of 'adverse reactions'. For definitions of what the different terms mean refer back to **What Are Allergies?**, page 7, and **When Is An Allergy Not An Allergy?**, page 15.

AVOIDING FOODS THAT COMPOUND YOUR ALLERGY PROBLEMS

Adverse reactions to foods are particularly common in the allergic condition. This does not mean that every allergic person has a problem with certain foods, but a large number do. You will not know which you are until you either attempt an elimination and reintroduction exercise, or have a blood test to see if that can give you some pointers. Allergy tests are most useful when there is a definitive IgE allergy to a food. Where there is an IgG reaction, the tests currently available are probably useful in about 70 per cent of cases (my estimation). The mechanism might not involve the immune system at all, but be a result of enzyme deficiency, meaning that compounds in certain foods cannot be processed properly, leading to adverse reactions which might be mistaken for allergies.

Elimination and reintroduction of foods, as long as it is carried out correctly, is the most reliable method of working out which foods are involved in adverse reactions. It is also the cheapest, because you can do it at home on your own, but it requires motivation, discipline and careful organisation. It involves totally avoiding the suspect foods for two weeks, and then reintroducing them in a controlled fashion, one by one, on different days, to ascertain which ones are the culprits. During this time a careful note should be kept of which symptoms disappear on avoidance, and which reappear on reintroduction. This method is suitable for the majority of people as long as a severe food allergy does not exist, such as anaphylaxis (see page 81) or brittle asthma (see page 128).

The most common foods involved in adverse reactions, and those that seem to compound allergy problems, are:

eggs
wheat-based foods
milk and other dairy products
soya
yeast
grains other than wheat, usually the gluten grains, rye,
   barley and oats
citrus fruit

peanuts
nuts, sesame seeds
deadly nightshade family: potatoes, tomatoes, peppers,
    aubergines
chocolate
pickled and preserved foods, such as salami
artificial food colourings

Other foods and drinks that also commonly contribute to allergy problems (though their negative effect is, at least in part, likely to be as a result of undermining the functioning of the immune system) include sugar, alcohol, caffeine, as well as smoking, recreational drugs and some prescription drugs. You must not stop taking prescribed medication without discussing this first with your doctor.

The appearance of a food on the above list does not mean that it is intrinsically bad. There is nothing wrong with citrus fruit, nuts, cheese, wholemeal bread, potatoes and tomatoes, for instance, unless you have a specific bad reaction to them. There is also nothing wrong with a little chocolate or the occasional coffee or sugary dessert, just so long as they are eaten in moderation and they do not cause adverse reactions. It is important not to become frightened of food when seeking to work out what is undermining your health, but to gain a sense of perspective and balance. Ways of dealing with eliminating these individual foods, including lots of alternative suggestions, are covered in the **Appendices**, page 135.

HOW TO TEST FOR ADVERSE REACTIONS TO FOODS

If you have a strong reaction to a given food, or foods, you may already know what is undermining your health. Most people, however, only have a vague idea, if any at all, of what may be troubling them. This is not surprising, since many foods to which people react are commonly eaten and may not result in a reaction until 72 hours later (see **When Is An Allergy Not An Allergy?**, page 15). This is why you need to be methodical about your investigations. If you are lucky, you will be one of the many people who react badly to the most common foods to cause trouble – wheat and/or dairy products. This may not seem at all lucky to you, because they are such staples in our lives. Nevertheless, it is a lot easier to uncover culprits such as these rather than the more obscure possibilities, plus there are now a tremendous array of foods and cookery books which make avoiding these staples considerably less of a problem than it once was.

So how do you work out what you need to suspect? The best way is to keep a food diary for a week and write down every morsel that passes your lips, including quantities. Be very specific and note down the ingredients of each meal. So, for example, instead of just 'ham salad sandwich', write down whether it was white, brown, wholemeal or pitta bread; whether you used margarine or butter; the quantity of ham; what the salad consisted of – lettuce, cucumber, tomato – and the type of dressing that was used. As you can see, the permutations for a simple ham sandwich are endless. Although you might think the bread is the obvious culprit, it might just as easily turn out to be the tomato.

It is often the case that the foods that cause problems are also the foods that we crave the most. If you find it hard to get through the day without, say, bread (or coffee or chocolate) then, frankly, that is where your suspicions should be directed. Because adverse reactions often involve frequently eaten foods, it is best to choose a time when you can concentrate on this exercise and spend some time investigating good alternatives to make the transition easier. (Attempting to do this at Christmas or other celebratory times is, therefore, likely to be bad idea.)

Check out the takeaway lunches available near your office, keep the refrigerator stocked with tasty snacks, keep individual portions of meals you enjoy handy in the freezer, and make a list of all the foods you *can* eat. If you always go out for a curry on a Friday night, decide which dishes will work for you; if you make yourself packed lunches, work out five options that are easy and which you enjoy; if you are likely to go round to friends' houses to eat, work out what your line is (allergy is a pretty good excuse for most people, and if they have seen you suffering in the past with asthma, eczema or hay fever they will usually be sympathetic). By working out in advance what you can do you will make your life a lot easier.

Once you know which foods you suspect, cut them out of your diet for a period of time, preferably a couple of weeks, though often a week can be sufficient. It is best to avoid all the foods you suspect you might be reacting to at the same time. This prevents confusion with reactions to one food masking that of another. Assuming that you have gained some relief from your allergic conditions, you can then reintroduce the foods one by one in a methodical way to see which foods trigger symptoms. You may get a reaction that is directly linked to your allergy, or you may get totally different symptoms, such as diarrhoea, stomach cramps or headaches. You must not, of course, reintroduce any foods to which you might have an anaphylactic reaction. You must also not follow this reintroduction programme without medical supervision if brittle asthma (the most severe form of asthma) is involved (see **Children and Allergies**, page 123).

Also keep a diary when reintroducing foods, to note what is going on and to avoid confusion. Eat a normal portion of food – that is a couple of slices of bread, a glass of milk, 85 g/3 oz of cheese, and so on. Only introduce one food a day – thus bread one day, pasta the next, milk after that, white cheese, yellow cheese, and so on. You may find that you react to one food and not the other, even if they are in the same 'group'. There are also different levels of sensitivity. Some people can tolerate a food perfectly well if they only eat it once or twice a week, while others cannot tolerate even the smallest amount, such as might be found in packaged food. This will obviously dictate how much you need to be a label-reader. It might be that the small amount of wheat found in the starch thickener used in a particular product is fine, and it is only a bowl of pasta that sets you off. Others may find that the small amount of starch thickener is sufficient to cause a problem.

Unfortunately, food labelling and food production methods are somewhat hit-and-miss affairs and even foods that say they are free of a substance, such as peanuts, have been found to contain traces. One of the reasons that those with dangerous allergies are often caught out is because manufacturers do not, at the moment, have to list the quantities of ingredients in a product. In addition, if a composite food is included, which makes up less than 25 per cent of the total product, such as sausagemeat on pizza, then the ingredients of this composite food do not need to be mentioned at all. It is also possible for traces of food to be left on manufacturing machinery, thus contaminating the next batch – so a nut free chocolate may be contaminated by a chocolate which included nuts on a previous run.

How quickly the effects of changes to the diet are felt depends on the person and the problem. Many people find immediate relief when they identify and eliminate problem foods. Others find it takes longer, perhaps a couple of weeks. In the case of rheumatoid arthritis fast relief might be gained, but it is more likely that the inflammation takes time to be dampened and it could take several weeks to three months. If hay fever is the problem no relief may be gained at all unless the measures are started well before the hay fever season. (See **A-Z of Allergies**, page 77.)

SUPPORTING YOUR IMMUNE SYSTEM

Your immune system is likely to be the key player in your allergy problems and supporting it, rather than undermining it, can only be of benefit. Avoiding foods that may be causing an adverse reaction is one of the first steps to take, so if you are doing this you are already a long way down the line. Stimulants are also responsible for suppressing the immune system. They might make you feel good in the short term, but in the long term they undermine your health. Stimulants are addictive, which makes them awkward to eliminate. If you need motivation to do this, it might help you to know that getting rid of them might mean that you can tolerate some suspected problem foods a little more often. Avoiding the use of excessive sugar, coffee, alcohol, cigarettes and other stimulants, for example, can improve your general health sufficiently for you to tolerate foods to which you were previously sensitive.

Antioxidants are vital for maintaining immune health and are key players in reducing allergic problems since they help to counteract the damage done to tissues (for instance the bronchioles in lungs) by free radicals, which the body creates as part of the allergic reaction. There is no substitute for getting at least five portions of fruits and vegetables daily, though I prefer 7–8 portions. This is not difficult to achieve if you make sure that you eat at least a couple of pieces of fruit with your breakfast, another couple of pieces as snacks throughout the day, and one portion of vegetables or salad with your lunch and two portions of vegetables with your evening meal.

Vitamin C is worthy of special mention in relation to the immune system and allergies, and its benefits alone should be enough to persuade you to eat the required number of fruits and vegetables, and possibly take a vitamin C supplement as well. It truly is a multi-faceted nutrient, being involved in:

- making white blood cells;
- building collagen, which strengthens mucus membranes and so keeps 'foreign bodies' at bay;
- anti-viral, anti-bacterial and anti-parasite activity;
- antioxidant activities, including enhancing the activity of other antioxidants, especially vitamin E;
- detoxifying histamine.

Most fruits and vegetables contain vitamin C, but some foods are richer in this nutrient than others, in particular citrus fruit, strawberries, blackcurrants, guava, fresh lychees, mangoes, papaya, peaches, brussel sprouts, cauliflower, kale, watercress, kiwi fruit, cabbage, broccoli and rosehip tea.

There are several herbs which can help build resistance and improve immune function. Two of the most effective and widely available are echinacea drops and devil's claw tea.

THE IMMUNE/DIGESTION LINK

One aspect of immune health that is often forgotten about is the importance of maintaining a healthy digestive system and bowel bacteria balance. You may think of your digestive tract as just a tube which deals with food, but it is actually the largest immune organ in the body. It is part of the 'front line' and ensures that, for the most part, friends rather than foes are absorbed into the bloodstream. Extensive and complex immune functions are going on all the time right there in the gut mucosa. By avoiding foods that cause adverse reactions you are already helping your gut carry out its immune functions more effectively. By following the advice which follows in **Nutrients Needed for Skin and Mucus Membrane Health** you will also be supporting the barrier and immune organ that is your digestive tract.

There is one other important factor in the relationship

between digestive health and the immune system. That is the balance of bacteria which live in the bowels. There are around 1–2 kg of bacteria inhabiting our gut walls, and they consist of about 400 different species. We actually have more individual bacteria in our bowels than we have cells in our bodies, and their health is crucial to our health. Some of the bacteria are 'friendly' and are necessary for:

- keeping the bowels mildly acidic, which is optimal for health;
- making certain nutrients – B-vitamins and vitamin K;
- killing off harmful bacteria by making natural antibiotics, and so supporting the immune system;
- producing butyric acid from dietary fibre to feed the cells of the digestive tract;
- helping in the final digestion of proteins and milk sugars;
- stimulating contractions of the walls of the bowels.

Other bacteria, however, are 'unfriendly' and if these get the upper hand the following occurs:

- levels of 'endotoxins' increase, which are a drain on the resources of the liver and the immune system, leading to a variety of symptoms, including headaches, skin problems and digestive problems;
- the beneficial bacteria are 'crowded out', which can allow the proliferation of food poisoning bugs as they have little opposition;
- the risk of diarrheoa and colitis is increased.

If you have been on repeated courses of antibiotics, have taken the pill for more than a year or so, have been under a lot of stress, have had a couple of pregnancies close together or eat a diet high in sugar or refined carbohydrates, you may well have an imbalance of bacteria since these are all things that can lead to, and perpetuate, the problem. Several things can be done to encourage healthy bowel bacteria that will support the immune system and reduce the likelihood of allergic reactions. These measures include:

● Ensuring that you get enough fibre in your diet. The foods to include on a regular basis (in other words at least one or two at every meal and snack) are whole grains, pulses and beans, fruit, vegetables, nuts and seeds.
● Supplementing fibre can help. Wheat bran is usually too aggressive for the digestive tract and using oat bran, rice bran, linseeds (flax seeds) or psyllium husks are better options.
● Eating plenty of live cow's, sheep's or goat's yoghurt (or live soya yoghurt), olive oil, garlic, onions, cabbage and Jerusalem artichokes encourages healthy bacteria.
● Taking live bacteria supplements that contain lactobacillus and bifido bacteria. If one brand does not have the desired effect, try another as they contain different strains of bacteria, some of which you might need more than others.

10 things that suppress your immune system
● excess alcohol
● a diet based on refined carbohydrates and high fat convenience foods
● food allergies and sensitivities
● smoking
● excess sugar
● stress (anxiety, tension, feelings of helplessness, depression)
● two or more pregnancies very close together

- recreational drugs
- a polluted environment (for instance too many chemicals in the home)
- excessive antibiotic use

10 things that boost your immune system
- laughter
- a minimum of five servings of fruit and vegetables a day – a serving being 80g
- regular exercise
- stable blood sugar levels, achieved by eating a wholefood diet
- drinking 2 litres of water daily
- meditation
- good bowel health – a fibre rich diet and live yoghurt help
- satisfying sleep
- a happy home and work life
- a daily antioxidant nutrient supplement containing vitamins A, C and E, and the minerals selenium and zinc

NUTRIENTS NEEDED FOR SKIN AND MUCUS MEMBRANE HEALTH

The skin and mucus membranes form a continuous barrier between our inner tissues and the outside world. All allergic reactions involve either the penetration of this barrier by an allergen or a reaction of this barrier to outside influences. The most obvious allergy reactions involving this barrier are those that involve the skin – eczema, hives or psoriasis. But all the others also involve this barrier: asthma involves inflammation of the mucus membranes inside the lungs; hay fever and sinusitis involve irritation of the mucus membranes inside the nasal and head cavities; colitis involves irritation of the mucus membranes of the lower bowel. In one sense, this makes treatment a little easier because the unifying factors to consider here are the building blocks that are needed for skin and mucus membrane health – no matter what the condition.

The cells of the skin and the mucus membranes are composed of proteins and fats. It is the fats that are of most interest to us, because the type of fats that are lodged in the cell membranes determine how flexible they are and what types of local hormones (prostaglandins) they manufacture. This in turn affects any inflammation (see below). I shall discuss essential fats in detail later, but for now it helps to remember that as well as having an effect on prostaglandins they also make up the actual structure of the cells themselves. They are powerful medicine indeed!

Certain other nutrients are vital for maintaining good skin and mucus membrane integrity. If the cells are well glued together and have strong membranes, they are less easily breached. This means that immune-challenging viruses and bacteria, as well as certain food allergens, have less chance of crossing the barrier and causing allergic havoc. For instance, if you have eczema a certain bacterium which resides on the skin surface has more chance of causing damage because eczema typically involves broken skin. The permeability of the gut wall can also influence how disruptive certain food allergens can be. Sealing those gaps and providing nutrients for skin healing therefore plays an important part in any nutritional approach to reducing the symptoms of allergies. In addition to the essential fats, the most important nutrients to consider are:

Vitamin A is an antioxidant vitamin essential for skin repair. Signs of deficiency include scaly skin, dry skin, acne, dandruff and other skin disorders. It is found in liver, fish oils, egg yolks, full fat dairy produce and oily fish. Beta carotene, found in dark green leafy vegetables and orange coloured vegetables and fruits such as apricots, carrots, pumpkin and mango, is converted in the body into vitamin A.

Vitamin C is a familiar antioxidant vitamin found in all fruit and vegetables, but particularly in citrus, strawberries, other berries, kiwi fruit, broccoli and cabbage. Vitamin C is needed for collagen synthesis and so is vital for the integrity and building of skin.

Vitamin E is an antioxidant vitamin that sits in themembranes of cells fighting off free-radical damage called lipid peroxidation. If the body lacks sufficient vitamin E (or vitamin C to support it), it leads to damage of the skin cells. Good sources are wheatgerm, vegetables oils, eggs, olive oil, nuts, seeds, whole grain cereals and brown rice. However, it is difficult to obtain large amounts of vitamin E from food.

Zinc is a mineral is needed for all protein growth processes, including the repair of skin and mucus membranes. More than 30 per cent of people do not get sufficient zinc in their diet. Good sources are nuts, pumpkin and sunflower seeds, red meat, liver, sardines, oysters, egg yolks, rye, tuna, berries and brown rice.

REDUCING INFLAMMATION

Because the nature of the human body is that it operates in a web-like fashion, you will already be doing a number of things that help to reduce inflammation. Avoiding foods to which you are sensitive is an important step and, as already mentioned, eating an antioxidant-rich diet is also vital in helping put out the inflammatory fire. In addition, there are two other essential steps that must be taken to help control the inflammation that is the main symptom of allergy:

- incorporating essential fats into your diet as often as possible, while simultaneously reducing your intake of damaging fats;
- supporting the adrenal glands to help them produce the natural steroid hormones which keep inflammation in check.

Understanding fats

Understanding the effects of dietary fats on the inflammation process, and putting this information to use, is one of the most important and fundamental means by which allergy problems can be either resolved or minimised.

There are three main categories of fats – saturated, mono-unsaturated and poly-unsaturated. In addition, there are hydrogenated fats, which are man-made but similar to saturated fats. It is members of the poly-unsaturated group that are responsible for making powerful anti-inflammatory substances in the body. It is this feature that makes them so important in the management of allergies.

Saturated fats are found mainly in animal produce. Sources of saturated fats include meat, poultry, full- and semi-skimmed milk, cheese, butter and lard. Saturated fats are a rich source of arachadonic acid, which in excess can stimulate inflammation (see below).

Hydrogenated fats are manufactured fats, not found in nature, that are made by adding hydrogen molecules back into unsaturated fats. The hydrogenation process effectively makes artificially-saturated fats (i.e. fats that are saturated with hydrogen molecules), and therefore they can be thought of as 'honorary' saturated fats. The configuration of these hydrogenated fats, which include the 'corrupted' fats, called trans-fats, means that they are not useful to the body and can block the processes of the useful unsaturated fats. In this way they also contribute to the problems of inflammation and have a close link to allergy problems. Hydrogenated fats are found in many margarines, as well as most processed foods. Unless a margarine claims to contain 'no hydrogenated fats' then it will almost certainly include them. If it doesn't contain hydrogenated fats, saturated vegetable fats will usually have been used in order to harden the normally liquid oils to make the margarine. There are a few exceptions to this rule and margarines which have been solidified by using emulsifiers (and which are therefore unsuitable for frying) will mostly preserve the unsaturated status of the oils used.

Mono-unsaturated fats have one hydrogen molecule missing from their structure. All fats contain a mixture of different types of fatty acids, and so mono-unsaturated fats will crop up in small amounts in many types of fats, but the oil that is the richest source of mono-unsaturated fat is olive oil. Diets that include large amounts of olive oil are known to be extremely healthy on many fronts. The mono-unsaturated fat found in olive oil is also sometimes referred to as omega-9. There are several reasons why it is a healthy option:

- By using olive oil, dependency on saturated fats and hydrogenated fats is reduced, which means that they cannot do as much damage;
- Olive oil is fairly heat stable, which makes it an excellent, and probably the best, choice for cooking;
- Extra-virgin olive oil, in particular, is a source of powerful

antioxidant compounds which are intrinsic to the olive – it's the dark green colouring which delivers these and lighter oils have less antioxidant benefit.

Poly-unsaturated fats have two or more hydrogen molecules missing from their structure – the number of hydrogen molecules missing, in which order and where, determines the type. There are many different types, but for our purposes the ones that are of the most interest are the two that are termed 'essential'. They are so described because we must get them from our diet, making them essential for our survival. Other unsaturated fats are capable of being made in the body, making them non-essential. The two essential fats belong to two different families of fats:

omega-3 fats which are mainly found in oily fish, flax seeds (linseeds), walnuts, pumpkin seeds, soya and hemp seeds and
omega-6 fats which are mainly found in vegetable, seed and nut oils, as well as in the nuts and seeds themselves. Because hydrogenated fats also have their starting point from these origins, even after they have adulterated, they are still referred to as omega-6 fats, though they do not have the physiological advantages of cold pressed, unprocessed oils.

I shall look in detail at these two essential fatty acids and their contribution in reducing inflammation later but, before I do this, it is necessary to become familiar with three other compounds, the prostaglandins, arachadonic acid and the leukotrienes.

Prostaglandins

The name 'prostaglandins' came about because they were first isolated from the prostate glands of bulls and the name has stuck.

We now know, however, that these biochemically active substances are manufactured in every cell in the body and that they have wide-ranging effects on body processes. More than 50 prostaglandins have been identified with a range of different activities, and (this is the important part) they are made from essential fatty acids.

The prostaglandins we are interested in can either have an inflammatory effect, which means that they contribute to the problem of allergies, or an anti-inflammatory effect, which means that they ease the problems of allergies. The prostaglandins that lead to inflammation if manufactured in excess are called PGE2, and the prostaglandins that subdue inflammation and allergic reactions are called PGE1 and PGE3. This is a summary of how they are made in the body:

PGE1 and PGE2

The first essential fat is called linoleic acid (LA) which is a member of the omega-6 family of fats. It is obtained from the diet from fresh nuts, seeds, their oils and vegetable oils. LA is converted by an enzyme called D6D (delta-6-desaturase) into a fatty acid called GLA (gamma-linolenic-acid). Many atopic people, however, have a block in the D6D enzyme and do not make this conversion adequately. Because the next stage after GLA can lead to anti-inflammatory prostaglandin manufacture, this block can mean that it is beneficial for some atopic people to skip the LA stage and supplement them directly with GLA (see chart below). GLA is then converted into DLGA.

DGLA can then go one of three routes:

1 It can be stored in cell membranes all over the body.
2 It can be converted into PGE1, which inhibits inflammation and enhances white blood cell performance in the immune system. PGE1 tends to be at low levels in allergic individuals.

3 It can be converted into arachadonic acid, which in turn can be converted into leukotrienes and PGE2, which tend to encourage inflammation, and certain substances, called thromboxanes, which encourage smooth muscle wall contractions (a problem for asthmatics) and blood clot formation.

Maintaining the correct balance between converting these fatty acids to PGE1 or arachadonic acid is very important in helping people with allergies.

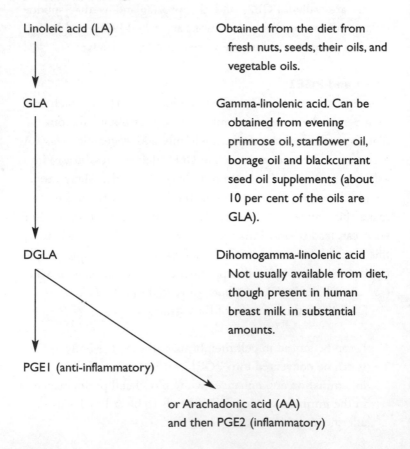

Linoleic acid (LA) Obtained from the diet from fresh nuts, seeds, their oils, and vegetable oils.

GLA Gamma-linolenic acid. Can be obtained from evening primrose oil, starflower oil, borage oil and blackcurrant seed oil supplements (about 10 per cent of the oils are GLA).

DGLA Dihomogamma-linolenic acid Not usually available from diet, though present in human breast milk in substantial amounts.

PGE1 (anti-inflammatory)

or Arachadonic acid (AA) and then PGE2 (inflammatory)

PGE3

The other essential fatty acid is ALA (alpha-linolenic acid) which is a member of the omega 3 family of fats. It leads to the other group of anti-inflammatory prostaglandins, the PGE3s. The way that we make PGE3 looks like this:

Alpha-linolenic acid (ALA) ↓	Obtained from some foods such as soya, walnuts, linseeds, pumpkin seeds and hemp seeds.
EPA and DHA ↓	Eicosapentanoic acid and Decosahexanoic acid. Apart from being made from ALA in our bodies they are also found in breast milk and are needed for the developing baby. Omega-3 deficiency can start early in life if the baby is bottle-fed. The highest concentrations of these two polyunsaturated fats are found in oily fish. As many people do not eat the foods in which ALA are found, this means that oily fish are their only source of these vital fats.
PGE3	As well as having an anti-clotting effect, reduces inflammation and is of tremendous therapeutic benefit for arthritis as well as for asthma, psoriasis, eczema and other allergies.

Converting essential fats

There are several factors which will inhibit the conversion of the essential dietary fats LA and ALA into the compounds which eventually make the anti-inflammatory prostaglandins. One of the enzymes responsible for these conversions, delta-6-desaturase (D6D), is fragile and can be inhibited by:

- low zinc and magnesium levels;
- smoking and alcohol;
- too many dietary saturated fats;
- too many dietary hydrogenated fats;
- high insulin levels, which usually result from high sugar levels;
- high stress levels.

It is also the case that many cases of atopic allergy are related to a genetic tendency to produce lower than normal levels of D6D. Because atopics have a lowered ability to metabolise omega-6 fats properly, this results in them having higher levels of arachadonic acid, the pro-inflammatory fatty acid. This increases their risk of allergic inflammation and results in the symptoms of allergies. It is incredibly useful, therefore, for these people to eat oily fish, which gives them EPA and DHA, and/or to take GLA supplements. By doing this they skip a stage of the conversion of the essential fats, and benefit from their therapeutic effects.

Arachadonic acid

Arachadonic acid (AA) is needed to promote wound healing as it encourages blood platelet stickiness; it is also important for nerve, brain and eye health. However, AA is not needed in vast quantities, and an excess of AA contributes to excessive inflammatory leukotriene production. For instance, people with psoriasis have elevated leukotriene levels in the affected skin. A natural source of high levels of AA is saturated fats found in animal produce, and an excess of animal fats can contribute to allergies because the AA they contain promotes inflammation. AA not only favours the synthesis of PGE2 but also of IgE immune cells involved in atopic allergy.

Omega-3 fats work competitively against AA converting into PGE2 (the inflammatory prostaglandin) by replacing the AA in cell membranes. However, from the time that you start eating more omega-3 fats, say by increasing your consumption of oily fish to 3–5 times a week, it is likely to take at least 18 weeks, possibly longer, depending on how many omega-3s you eat, for you to begin to notice the effects.

Leukotrienes

These are metabolites (end products) further down the line of fatty acid conversion. They have a number of different physiological purposes and effects, but some (those which follow on from arachadonic acid) are highly inflammatory and lead to some of the worst effects of allergies. The fish oils, and GLA, are effective at countering some of their worst effects.

Increasing levels of essential fats in your diet

There are some simple ways of making sure that your intake of essential fats increases, and that you decrease the non-beneficial fats that block their activity. Start to make the following changes, and in no time at all you will find that you have made significant alterations to the make up of your diet and begun to reap the benefit that healthy fats can have on your allergy problems:

- Replace at least three meat meals a week with oily fish such as mackerel, sardines, tuna, salmon, pink trout, pilchards, anchovies and shark. It is true that some people are allergic to fish, however, by far the majority of people, including those who are allergic, are not sensitive to fish and these people are likely to benefit greatly from including fish, particularly oily fish, in their diet on a regular basis.

- Make at least two meals a week vegetarian, based on pulses and beans.

- Snack on pumpkin seeds, sunflower seeds and fresh nuts such as walnuts and almonds. Keep these in the refrigerator, or in the freezer for longer-term storage.

- Use a tablespoon of cold-pressed flax oil to dress salads and vegetables (after they have been cooked) daily. Flax oil needs to be bought cold-pressed, in dark, preferably glass, bottles. It should be kept in the refrigerator and used within six weeks of opening and certainly before its sell-by date. If you buy it in bulk you can keep unopened bottles in the freezer to further prolong its freshness. The reason for all this effort is that flax-oil is very heat and light unstable, which is part of the reason why it is so biologically active, and therefore of use to our bodies.*

- Use nut butters or hummus on crackers and bread, instead of butter and margarine.

* It is a good idea to take an antioxidant supplement (vitamins A, C and E) at the same time as taking high doses of essential fats to reduce their oxidation in the body. In any event, antioxidants are vital for skin health, so there is a double benefit. Eating antioxidant-rich fruit and vegetables is also important.

Fish and plant oil supplements

You can take supplements of omega-3 and omega-6 fats as well as increasing levels in your diet. One of the commonest general remedies in the past was a dose of cod liver oil. Nowadays, it is usually advisable to take fish oil supplements rather than fish liver oil supplements because the latter can be contaminated with pollutants (though the best quality supplements have been cleansed). Flax oil is a good source of omega-3 fats if you are a vegetarian or vegan and do not wish to take fish oils, though for some conditions, such as arthritis and asthma, it is definitely the fish oils that have been proved in research to be of benefit. For conditions such as psoriasis, however, the flax oil is of equal benefit.

Essential fatty acid supplementation is not always straightforward. If you have a deficiency in omega-3 fats, which has built up over time, but not in omega-6s (or if an omega-6 excess exists) it can make the condition worse if you supplement the GLA omega-6 supplements (evening primrose, star flower, borage and blackcurrant seed oils). The best way forward, for most people, is to start with flax oil (from linseeds) and fish oils, to see if symptoms improve over two months. If they do not, suspect an omega-6 deficiency and take evening primrose oil or some other source of GLA.

If administering GLA supplements to small children, pierce the oil capsules and rub the contents into the skin, where they are well absorbed. This is of particular benefit in alleviating eczema and psoriasis, as well as being helpful for other conditions.

Evening primrose oil, and other sources of the omega-6s, should be avoided by those with epilepsy as they may worsen the condition. Those with bleeding disorders and those taking blood thinning medication need to check with their doctors before taking fish oil supplements as they can further thin the blood.

Supporting your adrenal function

All the measures discussed in **The Stress Factor**, page 4, are of importance in improving adrenal function. Many of the other measures I have discussed previously can also have an impact on adrenal health. For instance, identifying food sensitivities reduces the number of times your adrenal glands have to react to the 'emergency' of foods that disagree with your metabolism. Likewise, reducing or eliminating stimulants. The balancing of blood sugar levels that accompanies a low-stimulant diet also benefits adrenal health. Even changing the fats you eat has an impact, since the adrenal hormones are made from cholesterol, and eating healthy fats improves cholesterol production and balance. So, once again, if you have come this far, you have already done a lot of what is needed, since there is a compound effect to everything you do in relation to allergy problems.

All that is left is to identify which nutrients and herbs can be used to support adrenal function. There is definitely a case for taking supplements, in addition to addressing diet and stress levels, if your adrenal glands are tired and need a helping hand, the most useful being:

B vitamins are used for all energy production processes, and in particular B5 and B6 are used directly in the production of stress hormones. Food sources of the B-vitamins are whole grains, oatmeal, brewer's yeast, brown rice, legumes, liver, dark green leafy vegetables, egg yolks, molasses and yoghurt. Take a 50–100 mg B-complex supplement daily.

Vitamin C is the ultimate anti-stress nutrient. Normally excreted, the adrenal glands are the only store of this nutrient. It is needed in vast quantities to make stress hormones. Fruit and vegetables are our dietary sources, but you can also take 1–3 g daily (unless you are diagnosed with haemachromatosis).

Zinc is used for all repair jobs in the body and it is needed to make stress hormones. In addition to dietary zinc, take 15–25 mg daily. If you take an upper amount for more than three months, make sure your supplement has 1 mg copper for every 10 mg zinc.

Ginseng – the three ginsengs (Korean, Siberian and American) are all adaptogens. Adaptogens allow the adrenal glands to work more effectively and the body to 'adapt' to stress. Korean is the most stimulating, American the most calming and Siberian in between the two. Korean ginseng should not be taken if you have high blood pressure or breast disease.

Liquorice is an adrenal tonic (in its herbal, not candy form) and has cortisone-like effects which make it useful for inflammatory conditions. Do not use if you have high blood pressure, water retention or if you are taking steroids.

REDUCING YOUR HISTAMINE REACTION

Histamine is the chemical released by the mast cells lining the skin and mucus membranes when they are irritated by an allergen. The number of mast cells and their location largely governs what type of allergy a sensitive individual will suffer from. If large numbers of mast cells are lining the bronchioles of the lungs, asthma will result; if large numbers line the nose, hay fever is likely, and if large numbers are in the skin then hives can be a problem.

The first step in preventing a histamine reaction is to avoid the triggers which lead to the problem – you will probably know what these are for you, for instance tree pollen, cats or dogs, eggs, nuts, dairy foods, and so on. Another course of action is to avoid foods which are natural sources of histamine. These can add to the histamine 'load' and worsen reactions or trigger them themselves. These comprise mainly wine, beers and aged or fermented foods, such as salami or pickles. Some foods, a list of which appears in the Appendices, page 171, also have a histamine releasing effect. A histamine reaction to foods can seem similar to that of a true IgE allergy, but can be distinguished by the fact that relatively large amounts of the food are needed to trigger the histamine reaction, whereas only small amounts are needed to trigger an allergic reaction.

There are some natural antihistamine compounds that are helpful in reducing the histamine load and allowing the body to detoxify this powerful chemical. The best known of these is vitamin C. It needs to be taken in quite high doses of 1–3 g to have any effect, however, and some people will need 5 g daily. If taking this amount, it is much cheaper to buy powdered vitamin C, which is easily dissolved in water or juice. It is best to use a non-irritating type of vitamin C at these levels, such as magnesium ascorbate, sodium ascorbate, potassium ascorbate or Ester-C. The flavanoid quercitin has also been shown to have a histamine lowering effect and it works best if taken alongside vitamin C – the two enhance each other. Calcium at 500 mg daily helps to release histamine from the mast cells, thus enabling vitamin C to detoxify it. An amino acid (protein building block), methionine, also helps to process histamine out of the body.

You probably don't want to swallow so many supplements that you end up rattling, so when should you take them? They are most useful taken therapeutically. This means that if a histamine reaction is particularly bad for you, or if you know you are going away and are likely to have an allergic reaction to insect stings or bites, a three-month course of histamine lowering supplements may be of great use to you. If you are also addressing your diet, you will raise your general level of health and, hopefully, have a reduced allergic reaction in any event. This is not an absolute requirement for managing allergies, but a useful tool for times when it is needed. A three-month programme of daily supplementation would consist of:

3 g daily of vitamin C (taken in 3 divided doses)	also useful for many other aspects of managing allergy problems as well
500 mg of quercitin	helps to lower histamine reaction
500 mg of calcium	possibly as part of a multi-mineral supplement
500 mg of methionine	an amino acid which helps to metabolise histamine
50 mg B-complex	to balance the methionine

Another effective way of reducing histamine levels, and so helping with all allergic reactions is to take supplements of the reishi mushroom. Its anti-allergic and anti-inflammatory actions are due to the triter penoids it contains which inhibit key enzymes involved in inflammation.

CHAPTER SEVEN

Two-week Low Allergy Eating Plan

Allergies and food sensitivities are highly individual and, as a result, it is impossible to make a plan that suits everyone. However, this plan is a good way to start and should address a large number of problems for a large number of people

The plan has been designed to be high in essential fats, from oily fish, flax oil, nuts and seeds (those with the lowest allergy potential), as well as rich in antioxidants. This is to support the immune system and improve skin and mucus membrane health. The most common allergenic foods have been avoided: gluten grains (wheat, rye, oats, barley), dairy products (milk, cheese, yoghurt), soya, eggs, yeast (in breads, cheeses, beer and wine – though a small amount of vinegar and mushrooms are used) and peanuts. The levels of saturated fats from animal produce have been kept to a minimum, due to their inflammatory effects, as have levels of sugar. It is assumed that during this plan little or no alcohol, coffee or strong tea will be drunk (as a result you may experience headaches for a couple of days or so if you normally drink a lot of caffeine).

The plan is nutritionally complete, as long as you continue to eat a varied diet. If you find that it suits you, it can be followed as a blueprint for longer-term eating. Alternatively, you can use it to see if your symptoms resolve and, if they do, you can then slowly reintroduce foods into your diet to see if they result in a recurrence of reactions. For information on reintroducing foods see page 149. The foods that are most likely to be tolerated, and therefore should be reintroduced first, are soya products (such as milk, yoghurts and tofu), cow's yoghurt, barley, rye (crackers, bread), oats (oatcakes, porridge, oat milk), yeast-containing foods and peanuts and eggs (as long as you are not seriously allergic). After this reintroduce other dairy products such as milk and cheese and wheat-based products such as bread, cereals and pasta. Be methodical about how you reintroduce foods and, if you have any recurrence of symptoms, eliminate the foods again.

If this plan does not work for you, read the sections about your particular health problems in the chapter **A–Z of Allergies** and see the **Appendices** for rotation and elimination diets and other ideas of where to start looking for solutions to what ails you.

The plan is meant to be a celebration of food, not punitive. You may crave some foods that you commonly eat, but I hope that the eating plan is varied enough for you to enjoy it. It aims to give options for one easy meal a day (assuming that a packed meal can be taken to work) but, inevitably, it must be recognised that a reduced dependency on convenience foods may mean that more cooking than usual is involved. While many choices are given, in reality few people cook meals that are quite as varied as these. It is important, therefore, to develop the skill of planning ahead. Convenience lunches are in the plan – such as takeaway baked potatoes with fillings, dips from the deli counter and sushi. However, when it comes to some of the salads, for instance, or dishes such as chicken, onion and apple meatballs, you may need to prepare some of the ingredients the night before. This is quite easy and some meals, such as the meatballs, can be made and frozen ahead of time. Other ingredients, such as cooked millet grains or green beans, might constitute some of the previous evening's meal, with a portion left aside to add to a salad the next day. Ingredients such as chick peas or lentils are ideally cooked and kept in the freezer in portion sizes for when needed, but there is nothing wrong, from the point of view of allergies, in using a can instead. It is also a good idea to invest some time in buying in ingredients you might not have in your store cupboard, such as coconut cream and almond milk. Scout around your local supermarket, corner shop, ethnic shops and health food shop for other ideas of gluten- and dairy-free meals, in particular.

A number of vegetarian options are given, a few meat dishes, and several fish dishes – including some that use white fish for those who prefer it, although it is always best to use oily fish if you are able. Breakfasts have been repeated over the two weeks, with the exception of days 6 and 7 (the weekends) when you may have more time to prepare something a little more celebrational. Mix and match the ideas and dishes, there are no rules, the plan is highly flexible and can be adapted to your own needs.

Bon appétit!

WEEK I	BREAKFAST	EASY MEAL	MAIN MEAL	SNACK
DAY I	rice crispies with blueberries, strawberries and rice milk	baked beans on gluten-free toast tangerines	fishcakes made with potato or cooked millet, oily fish flakes and coated in rice flour (bind with rice milk) and served with assorted vegetables sliced oranges drizzled with honey and orange liqueur	Japanese rice crackers sultanas vegetable juice
DAY 2	gluten-free muesli (available from health food shops) soaked in apple juice overnight. Add grated apple before eating	takeaway fish or vegetable sushi strawberries and nut cream	Irish stew made with lamb, onions, root vegetables and millet, served with mashed potato or mashed swede halved, poached peaches filled with almond paste and toasted slivered almonds	walnuts pickled gherkins banana and peach wizz (made with rice milk)

WEEK I	BREAKFAST	EASY MEAL	MAIN MEAL	SNACK
DAY 3	millet porridge with rice milk, sliced banana and a little molasses or honey	thick lentil and vegetable soup sweet cured rollmop herrings with carrot sticks green and black grapes	polenta with roasted root vegetables and salmon melon balls with a tiny bit of ginger syrup	sunflower seeds dried apple rings prune juice
DAY 4	fruit compote with almond cream	tuna and sweet-corn salad with baked potato apple	large, fresh sardines grilled for five minutes (can be kept in freezer until needed) with tomato, olive and spring onion salad fruit salad with chopped dates and almond cream	almonds carrot sticks peach nectar
DAY 5	cornflakes with chopped papaya, raisins and rice milk	tortilla chips (wheat-free) with takeaway dip selection (hummus, salsa, guacamole) and crudités mango	Chinese take-away: rice, stir-fried broccoli with garlic, and squid baked banana sprinkled with cinammon	pumpkin seeds dried apricots apple juice

WEEK 1	BREAKFAST	EASY MEAL	MAIN MEAL	SNACK
DAY 6	potato rosti (grated potato and onion, patted into a cake and fried in olive oil) served with chutney	prawns, shredded lettuce, avocado and tomato salad with flax oil and balsamic vinegar dressing pineapple	poached salmon with celeriac purée and yam or parsnip chips strawberries dipped in dark chocolate	cashew nuts olives and cherry tomatoes tomato juice
DAY 7	bacon roll made with a gluten-free roll, lean bacon and chutney	chicken portion with pea and mint salad and coleslaw banana	stir-fried shredded vegetables with chestnuts, ginger and lemon grass served with quinoa lychees and star fruit	banana chips fresh coconut hot chocolate (made with rice milk)

WEEK 2	BREAKFAST	EASY MEAL	MAIN MEAL	SNACK
DAY 1	rice crispies with blue berries, straw-berries and rice milk	mixed salad: combine pre-washed salad, crudités, cooked chick peas and cooked buck-wheat, and serve with a flax oil and lime dressing pear	prawn and vegetable paella or prawn and vegetable pilau with papadums baked apple stuffed with dates and drizzled with coconut cream	Japanese rice crackers sultanas vegetable juice
DAY 2	gluten-free muesli soaked in apple juice overnight. Add grated apple before eating	green bean, tomato, onion and lentil salad with flax oil and olive oil vinaigrette dressing plums	fresh tuna baked with garlic, tomato, basil, pine nuts and balsamic vine-gar, served with rice noodles crystallised ginger	walnuts pickled gherkins banana and peach wizz (made with rice milk)
DAY 3	millet porridge with rice milk, sliced banana and a little molasses or honey	bean, tomato and basil soup anchovy tapenade with celery sticks two or three dark chocolate squares and raisins	burritos – corn tortillas with chicken, salsa and avocado filling mango ice (mash mangoes and chill in the freezer)	sunflower seeds dried apple rings prune juice

WEEK 2	BREAKFAST	EASY MEAL	MAIN MEAL	SNACK
DAY 4	fruit compote with almond cream	corn pasta salad with red peppers, olives and mackerel flakes, and an olive oil and lemon dressing orange	buckwheat pasta primavera (with lightly cooked broccoli, peppers, onions, asparagus or other vegetables in season) poached pears drizzled with raspberry coulis	almonds carrot sticks peach nectar
DAY 5	cornflakes with chopped papaya, raisins and rice milk	chicken, onion and apple meatballs served cold with salad banana	risotto made with wild mushrooms, asparagus and fresh peas (no parmesan), served with a crisp green salad chocolate covered almonds	pumpkin seeds dried apricots apple juice

WEEK 2	BREAKFAST	EASY MEAL	MAIN MEAL	SNACK
DAY 6	rice cakes with cashew nut butter topped with kiwi slices	aubergine paté (made by baking an aubergine in its skin, scooping out the flesh and blending it with tahini and lemon), served with rice cakes kiwi fruit	roasted monk-fish with grated ginger and rice-wine sauce, served with water-cress salad and orange slices poached figs with walnuts and almond cream	cashew nuts olives and cherry tomatoes tomato juice
DAY 7	pancakes made with gram (chick pea) flour and almond flour, served with nut butter, apple sauce and/or blue-berries	flaked tuna, red onion and white bean salad, served with a mixed leaves salad and an olive oil and flax oil dressing grapes	pheasant roasted with dried apricots and served with baked celery and millet (cooked like rice) baked rice pudding made with chopped nuts and coconut milk	banana chips fresh coconut hot chocolate (made with rice milk)

Part Four

A-Z OF ALLERGIES

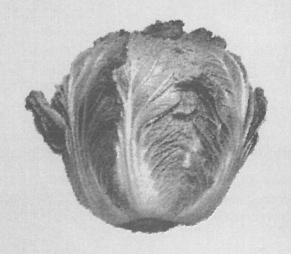

CHAPTER EIGHT

A-Z Of Allergies

Here specific problems have been organised in alphabetical order for ease of reference. Inevitably, there is some crossover between conditions, so it is possible to gain some insights by, for example, reading the section on hay fever, even though your problem is mainly asthma, or reading about eczema, even though the condition you want to treat is psoriasis.

There are some unifying factors of importance to almost all of these conditions, which have been discussed already in the previous chapter, **Strategies For Allergies**. These include bringing down inflammation by addressing essential fat and antioxidant intake in the diet, supporting the immune system and reducing the histamine reaction. Improving bowel health to increase the body's ability to get rid of toxins effectively (and to stop them contributing to skin problems and headaches) is also very important. Finally, a small reminder that for most of these conditions we are talking about skin or mucus membrane health and the factors which support the healing of these barriers are similar from condition to condition.

ALLERGIC COLITIS

The suffix '-itis' means a non-specific inflammation of an area of the body, thus colitis means inflammation of the colon. Colitis is characterised by diarrhoea, sometimes with blood and often with mucus in the stool, abdominal bloating and the need to go to the bathroom frequently. The degree of severity of symptoms is not necessarily related to the degree of inflammation or ulceration in the colon. Colitis mainly affects those in the 20–40 year age group, and it affects women more commonly than men. Inflammatory bowel disease is often confused with irritable bowel syndrome (IBS), however the term allergic colitis is increasingly being used to describe IBS in recognition of the fact that food allergies (or sensitivities) have a large part to play in the condition. Other factors also play a part, and stress, smoking and sugar consumption are common contributors to the problem. Most people will gain at least partial, and often total, relief from colitis and irritable bowel syndrome by investigating food sensitivities and avoiding certain foods. There is a tendency for colitis to recur in families, which suggests an atopic link, and there is also a higher incidence of eczema, hay fever and arthritic conditions amongst people with colitis.

The most likely causes of allergic colitis are:

- wheat-based foods and other gluten grains (see **Appendices**, page 154);
- dairy produce (see **Appendices**, page 152);
- aspirin – if this is the cause, a salycilate-free diet will, in rare cases, resolve the condition (see **Appendices**, page 172).

It can also help to avoid foods that can irritate the bowel if you are susceptible. These include curries, strong spices, chilli, coffee and strong tea. A diet which features too much sugar is also counter productive.

It is also very important with any bowel problems to take a supplement containing beneficial bacteria. Our bowels are home to billions of micro-organisms, some of which are essential for our good health. If there is any bowel disturbance, as often happens with allergies but particularly with allergic colitis, normalising the bowel bacteria can have great benefits. Research has confirmed that supplementing lactobacilli bacteria lowers the incidence of diarrhoea and improves immune tolerance to food antigens. A good beneficial bacteria supplement will contain at least one billion viable organisms per capsule, and needs to be kept refrigerated and taken before the use-by date. Adults need to take a combination of lactobacilli and bifido bacteria. Children should take bifido infantis until they are one or two years of age, and then switch to the adult bacteria (you cannot overdose on these bacteria, though see paragraph that follows about other ingredients in the capsules).

Supplements containing lactose, FOS (fructo-oligo-saccharides) or other sugars can make the condition worse. FOS is actually beneficial to use in the long term, as it promotes the growth of beneficial bacteria, however it can lead to unpleasant symptoms of gas in the short term, when doses of over 1 teaspoon are taken by people with very sensitive bowels. Other fibres can also make the symptoms worse if suddenly introduced into the regime, however, taking half a teaspoonful of psyllium husks and building up to one or two teaspoons, very slowly over time, is a very gentle and non-irritating way of encouraging healthy bowels (though if it aggravates the condition at all you must cut back the dose immediately).

Herbs such as slippery elm, aloe vera and meadowsweet have also been shown to encourage healing of the mucus membranes in colitis.

For more information about digestive disorders see *Banish Bloating* in this series of books.

ANAPHYLAXIS

Anaphylaxis is the most severe type of allergy. In its worst form, a serious allergic reaction can occur which involves the swelling of tissues, mainly around the mouth, face and throat. If left untreated, it can lead to suffocation as the breathing tubes close up. There may also be severe asthma, shock and unconsciousness and even death. It is extremely serious and should never be taken lightly. At the first sign that someone is having an anaphylactic reaction, even if it is mild and just involving tingling of the lips and tongue, they should immediately be taken to the nearest doctor's surgery, or the emergency services should be called if it is anaphylactic shock. A syringe of adrenaline will be administered which is life-saving. There is very little time to spare in the case of anaphylactic shock, and speed is of the essence. People known to be at risk can be prescribed pre-loaded adrenaline syringes for self-treatment.

The term anaphylaxis was first coined by the French scientist Charles Richet in 1903. He was aiming to immunise his dog against poisoning by jelly fish by giving it repeated injections. Treatment given in anticipation of a problem is called prophylaxis, but his dog suffered exactly the opposite effect on being given the second injection and died – so this reaction was called anaphylaxis. The first exposure to the allergenic food or substance is the one where the immune reaction is being 'programmed' and the second one is when the reaction starts to manifest.

If you are very unlucky, a severe reaction will take place on the second exposure to a food or substance, and while this is very rare it is also extremely serious. Subsequent reactions are difficult to predict, but it should be assumed that they may be just as severe, or even more so. Your case should be assessed thoroughly by a medical allergist.

When introducing your child to new foods, be aware of those which most commonly cause allergic reactions, particularly if there is a history of allergies in your family. Think how you would get to a doctor quickly in the event of a reaction occuring. The highest risk foods are: peanuts, tree nuts, sesame seeds, shellfish, eggs, milk, soya and fish, though any food could be a culprit, including fruit. It is not uncommon for wheat flour to be contaminated with dust mites, and it is possible for those with respiratory allergies to have an anaphylactic reaction to them. Storing flour in the refrigerator reduces this problem.

Anaphylactic symptoms in children can include abdominal pain and vomiting and in people of all ages could include a swelling of the lips, tongue and face, a generalised rash, shortness of breath, falling blood pressure or a loss of consciousness.

Anaphylaxis can occur as a result of allergy to a number of compounds and foods. Common triggers are wasp and bee stings, drugs including antibiotics and certain foods. These are usually lifelong allergies which means that it is essential to avoid exposure to the offending substance. If you have been prescribed adrenaline this will need to be carried at all times for emergency treatment, and you might also want to wear a Medic Alert bracelet which gives information about hidden conditions in case you fall unconscious. There is a surprising lack of awareness amongst sufferers of the need to carry these syringes and, even now, several deaths happen each year.

It is difficult for the allergic person to know if they are going to be exposed because of food labelling and production inadequacies mentioned previously. It is possible for someone to be so hypersensitive that even the molecules of food floating in the air near them can be sufficient to trigger a reaction, and a case was reported recently of a girl who died as a result of just being in the same room as an open jar of peanut butter. Severely allergic people need to be extremely watchful about food prepared in restaurants, as the chefs may not understand the true importance of cross contamination of foods, and they may also need to carry their own meals on to planes. The link between the food to which you are allergic, and the food you are eating, is not always obvious. Sarah, the daughter of David Reading, who started the Anaphylaxis Campaign in the UK, died after eating a lemon meringue pie in a restaurant of a well-known chain because she was unaware that it contained crushed peanuts.

It is never wise to test for the presence of an ingredient to which you know you are severely allergic by having a small taste, as a reaction can always be severe, even if it was milder the previous time.

In some cases, anaphylaxis is only brought on by a combination of the problem food followed by exercise. No reaction is provoked by exercise after fasting or after an allergen-free meal, nor by eating the allergens and avoiding exercise. In one medical report, foods as diverse as tomato, courgettes, wheat, potato, peanuts and rice caused reactions once the individuals exercised, and these allergies were also confirmed by RAST (see **Allergy Tests**, page 178).

It is also common for an allergy to antibiotics to develop, so all patients should be asked before a course of treatment if they know whether they are allergic to them. Allergies can develop to any drugs, including anaesthetics and vaccines, as they can to most other substances. If you are allergic to antibiotics, your doctor should be able to prescribe a different class of antibiotics to the ones to which you are known to be allergic. The best policy, if you know that you have an allergy problem to specific antibiotics, is to avoid the need to use them. This means supporting your immune system and its natural ability to fight off bacterial infections, and using immune enhancers and natural antibiotic compounds such as garlic, echinacea, grapefruit-seed extract, goldenseal and St John's wort. It is doubly important to use beneficial bacteria supplements to improve your response to bacterial infections. Of course, if a serious infection sets in, you must always refer to your doctor for evaluation. Measures for supporting your immune system are discussed on page 45.

ARTHRITIS

There are so many factors involved in arthritis management that it is really the subject of a separate book. However, a significant number of people benefit from following advice for dealing with food allergies and sensitivities, so here I will simply look at the role that these can play on the condition. In osteo-arthritis, nutritional intervention (including treatment for food allergies and using antioxidants and fish oils) can help to limit inflammation that results from the wear and tear that is typical of the condition, but these have a limited effect on the under-lying condition. In the case of rheumatoid arthritis, however, many people find significant relief and reversal of their symp-toms by changing how they eat. Because the immune system is involved in the condition of rheumatoid arthritis (RA), it seems that diet can have a direct modulating effect on the course of the disease.

While avoiding certain foods can have a fairly rapid result when seeking to resolve many allergy or food intolerance problems, it can take quite a lot longer for RA. Sometimes it is necessary to embark on an exclusion diet for at least 12 weeks before you even begin to start to feel a difference. This means that a certain amount of dogged determination is needed. It is also true that if you slip during that time, a lot of the good can be undone as the body often becomes hypersensitive and reacts badly. On the bright side, some people respond much quicker, and you may be one of them!

The main suspect foods as far as RA is concerned are all wheat-based products, all dairy products, all citrus fruit and all members of the deadly nightshade family – tomatoes, aubergines, sweet peppers, hot peppers and potatoes (though sweet potatoes are fine to eat, and see **Appendices**, page 151 for other alternatives). At the same time, cut out smoking (tobacco is also a member of the nightshade or belladonna family) and all alcohol and sugar. I hear you groan, but it is possible and can be very rewarding. At the end of a 12-week period many RA sufferers find relief and can experiment, slowly, with reintroducing the foods one-by-one to determine which ones have an adverse effect. I cannot stress enough how important it is with this condition to start by eliminating all of these foods at the same time. The same results are usually not achieved by cutting them out one at a time.

It is worth mentioning two case histories here to provide extra motivation. One lady, who had been crippled with RA since childhood, was in such a bad state that, as a young woman, she was almost totally dependent on her mother to do such things for her as combing her hair and helping her in the bathroom. At a later date her husband took over this role. She was determined to help herself, however, and underwent many treatments, both orthodox and complementary. Finally she addressed her diet in the way described above, though she did not give up the couple of glasses of wine which she found a great comfort at the end of the day (she was by now in her fifties). She can vouch for the difference this regime made to her comfort and mobility – she even managed to take up sailing as a hobby! The only time she lapsed was when she was occasionally tempted by a brie baguette (her favourite) and then she paid for it with a couple of days of severe swelling and discomfort. Other than this, she was able to more or less control her symptoms and described them as 80 per cent improved. I managed to convince her to go the last mile and to experiment with avoiding alcohol for only one week. She was amazed at the difference that just this one extra step made to her comfort levels and is happy to continue with avoiding alcohol for the time being. I suspect that she may want a glass of wine from time to time but, as with the baguettes, she knows what the consequences will be and will make a judgement about whether it is worth or not – she is in control.

Another lady with RA, whose story stands out in my memory, adopted all the recommended measures and, true to form, it took about three months for her to feel any benefit, but she eventually gained great relief. Her husband, who was very supportive, decided that he was going to go on the regime with her. He had been having to go to his doctor weekly to have his blood pressure checked, as it was dangerously high. While she struggled on for 12 weeks before seeing any result, he found that within a couple of weeks his blood pressure had come down dramatically, to the astonishment of both himself and his doctor, so you never know who will be helped by these changes!

There isn't space here to go into the subject of arthritis any more than this, other than to say that fish oils can benefit the condition significantly by helping to change the factors that lead to inflammation, and antioxidant vitamins and minerals are also of paramount importance. In addition to eating plenty of oily fish (such as mackerel, sardines, tuna, salmon, anchovies, pink trout and pilchards) and fresh fruit and vegetables, and cutting back dramatically on saturated fats from meats, cheese, full fat milk and butter, I would also advise any person with arthritis to make sure they take fish oil supplements, possibly flax oil as well, and a high-dose antioxidant supplement.

ASTHMA

Not many things can be as bad as gasping for the very breath of life and feeling that you might not be able to. It is excruciating to watch an attack happening, especially if it is a child who is suffering. The lungs are delicate and vulnerable organs and the oxygen that filters through them is our most important nutrient – we die after only a few minutes without oxygen.

Asthma is a disorder of breathing characterised by narrowing of the airway within the lung. The main symptom is breathlessness and inflammation is the main underlying cause. Getting this under control is a major factor in treatment, as well as finding what triggers are involved.

The wheezing of asthma can develop in childhood, but also in adult years. Childhood asthma may be preceded for several months, or years, by episodes of coughing, slow recovery from upper respiratory tract infections, which later develop into bronchitis and eventually asthma. The risk of childhood asthma is increased by parental smoking, and by antibiotic usage by the child in the first year of life. Conversely, a study of 2,400 children noted that cat and dog exposure in the first year of life reduces the likelihood of asthma (probably because of the ability to build up immunity). Breast-feeding for longer than four months also reduces the incidence, as well as that of other allergies.

Adult asthma is more common in women than in men, and there may be obvious triggers which set off an attack – or there may not be. Even if there are known triggers, it is possible for others to develop later on. There are a number of possible triggers of asthma, but the end result of all types is the same, with the smooth muscle in the bronchioles (the lungs airways) becoming inflamed and producing mucus making breathing very difficult. In the worst cases it can be life threatening. One under-reported fact is that the majority of people who die from anaphylaxis are also asthmatic, and it is the asthmatic attack that follows the allergy reaction which kills them.

Some common triggers of asthma
- inhaled allergens such as house dust mites, animal dander, pollens, mould spores
- irritating gases, including cigarette smoke

- ingested allergens, including foods, drugs (including aspirin and coloured medicine coatings and syrups), food additives, yeasts in foods and moulds found on foods
- chemicals found in household products and in the work-place
- temperature changes, especially going from warm to cold air
- changes in the weather, including thunderstorms, since the weather may affect levels of pollutants, dust or moulds
- viral or bacterial infections
- exercise, sometimes only when combined with another trigger
- emotional stress

Asthma is now viewed as an ailment of affluence. It apears to be more likely to affect those who come from cleaner homes and smaller families, as they are less exposed to the germs that may help the developing immune system to build up its defences. Antibacterial cleaners, for instance, while they may protect from acute illnesses, kill off bugs so effectively that they make the environment at home too sanitised if overused.

Conversely, over furnished houses are also likely to be contributing to the problem, with carpeting and soft furnishing acting as home to billions of house dust mites. In the UK, asthma capital of the world, 98 per cent of homes have fitted carpets, compared to 16 per cent in France and only 2 per cent in Italy. Up to 100,000 dust mites can live in one square yard of carpet, each producing 20 droppings a day. It is the droppings that are the irritant for most people with asthma. Conventional vacuuming and washing has little effect on the levels of drop-pings in the carpets. Reduced ventilation, smoky atmospheres and increased humidity in homes also play their part in trigger-ing asthma, as do strong scents. Three-quarters of asthmatics react to people wearing strong fragrances and to other products such as 'fresh-air' products (see **The Pollution Factor**, page 31). On the subject of fresh air, if you smoke in the house it increases the likelihood of asthma for the non-smokers and children in the family.

The presence of a known and definite inhaled allergen does not preclude the possibility of other triggers, particularly ingested allergens. The most common food allergens for asthmatics are cow's milk, eggs, wheat, artificial colourings, cheese, yeast and fish, though almost any food can be a trigger. The asthmatic reaction to a food can be immediate, which makes it easier to detect, but it often also follows the pattern of delayed reaction described earlier. It is not always clear what the actual trigger may be so, for example, wine may cause an asthma attack, but it could be the yeast in the wine or the metabisulphate used as a preservative in wine production.

A diet for asthmatics needs to follow all the principles for avoiding inflammation, cutting out excessive saturated fats, fried foods, cured meats and hydrogenated fats (replacing them with unsaturated fats).

Studies have shown that the oils found in fish are particularly helpful to asthmatics. When an asthma attack happens, the reaction produces leukotrienes called LTB4 and LTC4. It is these substances that lead to the breathlessness and discomfort associated with asthma. The omega-3 fats found in oily fish significantly reduce the production of these irritants and so improve lung function. Leukotrienes that lead to the inflammation in asthma are 1,000 times more potent and irritating than histamine, and the omega-3 fish oils have the ability to block their formation. In various studies, canned fish and non-oily fish (white fish) were found not to be protective, but fresh oily fish, and fish oil supplements, really did make a difference. Children who eat oily fish have significantly less asthma. The length of time it takes to see results from when you start eating oily fish regularly is probably at least 18 weeks.

Other types of fats have been found to worsen the incidence of asthma, as well as conditions such as rhinitis and conjunctivitis. The high omega-6 content of many cooking oils, for example sunflower and corn oils, as well as the hydrogenated fats found in margarines and many commercial packaged foods, are at fault. It is better to cook with olive oil and to avoid margarines that use hydrogenated fats.

Theoretically, GLA fats found in evening primrose oil, borage oil, blackcurrant seed oil and starflower oil, can make asthma worse in some cases, in particular where there is already an excess of omega-6 fatty acids in the system (see **Fish and plant oil supplements**, page 61). For this reason it is probably wise to avoid these if you suffer from bad asthma attacks, and at least be aware of the possibility if your attacks are milder. They do not have the proven track record of improving the situation for asthmatics that fish oils do.

Athsmatics are often unable to take aspirin, as it can trigger an attack, so the painkiller of choice is usually paracetamol. Yet even a moderate intake of paracetamol has been shown to increase the risk of asthma developing, probably because the drug compromises liver health, leading to a reduced ability to deal with air pollution.

Avoid sulphur-based preservatives in dried fruit, dehydrated vegetables (i.e. instant potato or packet soup), mushrooms, desiccated coconut, peeled potato products, processed meats, vinegar, grapes, grape juice, wine, beer and cider. Until the practice of using sulphur preservatives on salads in restaurant salad bars was stopped, it was fairly common for them to trigger severe attacks in asthmatics.

The antioxidants found in fruit and vegetables are of particular benefit to asthmatics and help to protect against the effects of oxidation damage to the lungs and the build up of environmental toxins on the body in general. A vitamin C-rich diet, in particular, has a good association with lowered asthma incidence. Antioxidants help to reduce inflammation and to get rid of pollutants, such as lead, which may be involved in contributing to asthma. The flavonoid quercitin found in apples has been demonstrated to improve lung health, and it seems that an apple a day has more value for supporting the mucus membranes, lung function and lung capacity than eating many other fruits. The proanthcyanidin antioxidants found in dark berries, such as cherries, blueberries, raspberries, blackberries and elderberries are also potent lung-specific aids. In winter, frozen or canned berries have just as much value as fresh berries, though make sure you buy fruit canned in natural juices and not in syrup or sugar. Alternatively you could make a cordial made up of 80 per cent fruit and 20 per cent fructose (fruit sugar).

If you decide to give up coffee as part of a health regime, perhaps to avoid insomnia or digestive problems, you may find that your asthma attacks get worse instead of better. This is because caffeine is similar to theophylline (which is also present in coffee), a compound that is of proven therapeutic benefit to asthmatics. Caffeine, in my opinion, generally undermines good health, but there may be a case for asthmatics not to give it up too suddenly, but to reduce intake over time.

Some studies have shown a vegan diet to be highly effective at getting rid of the problem of asthma. It takes a certain mindset which will not suit all people, but if you think that this is for you, a carefully constructed vegan diet may be a good thing. Veganism avoids all animal products, including meat, poultry, fish, eggs, dairy produce and butter. If well managed, there is no reason to end up deficient in nutrients, though it is wise to take a multi-nutrient supplement which gives B12, vitamin D, vitamin A, zinc and iron. If you wish to embark on this sort of diet, it is advisable to read a good book on the subject first. To the best of my knowledge, there are no studies on people who deal with their asthma by following a vegan diet while also eating oily fish (which is, of course, a contradiction in terms), but this might be even more beneficial and more manageable.

Asthma has also been linked to high salt levels in the diet, but other trials where salt was specifically excluded or included have not borne this out. It is possible that high general levels of salt intake are also linked to other dietary factors such as hydrogenated fat or sugar consumption from a diet based on too many processed foods.

Some specific nutrients can be effective at reducing the number and severity of asthmatic events, by blocking or interfering with the metabolism of chemicals that trigger attacks. Vitamin B6, 50–100 mg daily, can help to reduce the level of even severe asthma, even in asthmatics who take steroids (do not stop taking your steroids as prescribed). Apart from B6, also take a B-complex supplement which gives 10–20 mg daily. Flax oil (1–2 tablespoon daily), zinc (10–20 mg daily), vitamin C (500–1,000 mg daily), vitamin E (600 ius daily) and selenium (100–200 mcg daily) can all help to reduce symptoms, but obviously have their best effect when dietary changes are made as well. You can get the majority of these nutrients in a high dose multi-supplement. Other useful supplements might be magnesium citrate (200–300 mg daily) which is a muscle relaxant, beta-carotene 20,000–25,000 ius (12–15mg) daily to support the mucus membranes of the lungs, and the bioflavonoid quercitin.

Liquorice root is a herb of value to asthmatics. It has a similar structure to cortisone, which is produced by the adrenal glands, and has an anti-inflammatory action. Unlike cortisone drugs, however, it doesn't atrophy the adrenal glands. It also helps to stabilise blood sugar levels. Do not, however, take liquorice root if you have high blood pressure, and if you use it regularly you need to make sure that your diet is high in potassium from fruit and vegetables, as it has the effect of increasing elimination of this mineral.

MSM (methyl sulfonyl-methane) is a naturally occurring sulphur compound, found in breast milk and very fresh produce, which is now available in supplement form. It helps the detoxification process and many asthmatics swear by it. It is also helpful for hay fever and other respiratory and lung problems.

Artificial colours in foods should always be avoided if possible. Children are particularly exposed to them as they are used liberally in child-appeal drinks, sweets and desserts, such as jellies. The azo dyes in particular, such as sunset yellow and carmoisine, have been found to be a problem. See **Appendices**, page 168.

While sudden exercise can trigger an asthma attack in some individuals, regular physical exercise may actually reduce the tendency towards asthma in general. Swimming in a warm, indoor pool, seems to be particularly beneficial for children. If you suffer from exercise-induced asthma, taking a high dose of vitamin C (1 teaspoon powdered vitamin C, or 5 g) half an hour before exercise can reduce the likelihood of an attack because it lowers levels of histamine. The herb ginkgo biloba may also be useful, possibly because it improves circulation to the area.

Stressful situations can trigger an asthma attack, particularly when they have been associated with asthmatic problems in the past. Avoiding situations that you know are stressful for you is obviously therefore important (see **The Stress Factor**, page 25).

Chamomile is very soothing for asthmatics and an infusion can be taken a few times a day. It is also effective when used as a steam inhalant. Asthmatics need to be careful about what they inhale, and aromatherapy oils should not be used, except under expert guidance.

Many women find that their asthma worsens pre-menstrually. Addressing food sensitivities, particularly wheat, sugar and caffeine intake can make significant inroads into pre-menstrual problems. Essential fats have a beneficial effect on both PMS and asthma, as does magnesium supplementation at 300–600 mg daily. The Harvard Nurses Study of 23,000 women has thrown up the statistic that those on HRT were 50 per cent more likely to have adult-onset asthma. Women generally have more asthma risk than men, in part because it is linked to oestrogen, which of course HRT carries on providing beyond the menopause. Another course of action that might yield results for you is to practice a breathing technique called the Buteyko method, which originated in Russia (see **Resources**, page 185).

Please also read the information regarding brittle asthma in the chapter on **Children and Allergies**, page 123.

ECZEMA

The term eczema comes from the Greek *ekzeein*, meaning 'to boil over', a fair description in severe cases when blisters ooze. Eczema typically manifests itself as dry, red, inflamed, itchy skin eruptions that sometimes also have small bubbles just under the skin surface which, in weeping eczema, erupt on the surface and can become infected. Eczema is not contagious. The term dermatitis is mostly interchangeable with the word eczema, though it usually means that the skin irritant is from an external source.

Treatment of these skin conditions usually involves steroid creams applied to the area but, while these can subdue the immediate inflammation, they do not do anything to prevent the problem recurring, and in fact can lead to a worsening of the condition in the long run as the skin can become thinner and more fragile from using them. The skin is a mirror of our inner health, and many skin conditions can successfully be treated by paying attention to diet and to nutritional deficiencies.

Contact dermatitis or eczema

Exogenous eczema is caused by external factors and is an irritated or allergic response to skin contact with various substances. This is a common cause of eczema and, while it is obvious to the person that something externally is triggering the problem, they are not always certain what this something is. The usual culprits are perfumes, washing powder, a plant, a metal (such as nickel in jewellery or belt buckles), items of clothing or other sources of chemicals (such as chlorine in swimming pools or solvents).

Use gloves and other protection when you know you might come into contact with something to which you are sensitive. In addition to avoiding known external allergens, supporting your immune health and making sure that you do not have any nutritional deficiencies (particularly in those nutrients involved in skin health – zinc, essential fats and vitamin A), can improve the situation, make you less sensitive to the trigger and help ensure, if you do react, that you heal more quickly.

It is a good idea with all eczemas to use non-biological washing powder, wear cotton clothing, particularly underwear, use cotton bedding, and avoid synthetics and wool, both of which can exacerbate the problem.

Seborrhoeic dermatitis and discoid eczema

These are the least common forms of eczema. Seborrhoeic dermatitis is a mildly itchy, red, scaly and greasy rash, which is usually found on the oily parts of the skin around the nose, the chin and the forehead, behind the ears, on the chest, between shoulder blades, in the armpits, in the groin and under the breasts in women. B-vitamin deficiency is often involved in seborrhoeic dermatits, particularly of vitamin B6. Taking a strong B-supplement of around 100 mg daily, plus one or two tablespoons of cold-pressed flax oil daily, avoiding refined carbohydrates and sugar, reducing intake of animal fats, identifying food sensitivities, and possibly food colourings, can all make a difference. It can also help to come off the contraceptive pill. Discoid (nummular) eczema affects adults and is often stress related. It appears as coin-shaped patches that look similar to ringworm, usually on the arms, legs and trunk.

Atopic eczema

Atopic eczema, otherwise known as endogenous or allergic eczema, is linked to over-sensitivity to common environmental factors, such as allergy to certain foods or to house dust mites (which are involved in 85 per cent of adult eczemas). Eczema is common in children, but also occurs with great frequency in adults. It is often triggered by events such as pregnancy and breast-feeding. The increased need for essential fatty acids and zinc during pregnancy and breast-feeding, both of which nutrients are also required for skin health, probably contributes to eczema developing at this time.

Typically, atopic eczema appears in children before the age of four, and then settles down a bit, before flaring up again at puberty. After that it may get a bit better, but have a tendency to flare up again. In children it is often the case that eczema develops when the child is weaned from breast milk to formula cow's milk, or to cow's milk in the diet. Breast-feeding for six months or ideally a year, thereby delaying or avoiding the introduction of formula milk, as well as avoiding the common triggers when weaning (milk, eggs, soya, oranges) can reduce the risk of your child developing eczema in the first place. Ten per cent of children with eczema also have both asthma and hay fever.

The first thing to exclude is the possibility of contact dermatitis. After this investigate the question of food allergies and sensitivities. It is almost always the case that those with eczema have some nutritional deficiencies, in particular zinc and essential fatty acids. Magnesium is another mineral which is almost always deficient if there is an allergy reaction and supplementing it can lead to improvements. These nutrients are notoriously depleted by chronic stress. Stress management is important because 60 per cent of sufferers link flare-ups to stressful events. The problems also often become worse in winter, probably because of a combination of cold winds, less sun, excessively heated rooms and possibly less antioxidants in the diet from fruit and vegetables.

Recent research has suggested a link between the intensity of the flare-up with a type of bacteria found on the skin, *Staphylococcus aureus* (SA), which is one of the antibiotic resistant superbugs. Ninety-five to 100 per cent of children with eczema have been found to have SA, while children without eczema do not seem to have it – and the worse the eczema the greater the concentration of SA. The suggestion is is that they are probably allergic to the toxins produced by the SA and, because the skin is broken, the super-antigenic exotoxins get through. Logic dictates that if the skin is provided with the nutrients it needs to help repair itself, the problem might be reduced. Maintaining the pH of the skin also plays an important part in helping the balance of the bacteria on the skin to rectify itself. The skin is covered in billions of bacteria, some beneficial and some detrimental, but the beneficial ones are encouraged by keeping the skin at the correct pH of about 5.7 acidity. Soap strips the acidity, whereas there are several skin washes and other products available that are based on being at the correct pH. Remember, however, that if a product has a neutral pH this is still, at 7.0, too alkaline, and it is the 5.5–5.9 range that is ideal. You can use the herbal tinctures of echinacea or goldenseal, diluted in water, as an anti-bacterial face wash. Tea tree oil is also a good anti-bacterial and can be applied by dabbing on with cotton wool.

Twenty per cent of adult eczemas are linked to a yeast on the skin, *Pityrosporum orbicular*, which leads to scurf, a flaky skin deposit. Your doctor can prescribe an antifungal cream, which is probably the quickest way of dealing with this problem, or you can use natural antifungals such as tea tree oil or grapefruit seed extract applied with a cotton pad. It also helps to avoid reinfection if you follow a low-sugar, low-yeast diet (for sources of yeast in foods see **Appendices**, page 159).

Many foods can help resolve the problem of eczema. As already mentioned, antioxidants are vital for skin health and a diet rich in fruit and vegetables is a key therapeutic tool. Making fresh juices and smoothies is a delightful way to get lots of antioxidants. Taking a daily antioxidant supplement is also beneficial. Foods that are rich in eczema-beating compounds include carrots, sweet potatoes, apricots, pumpkin, parsley, pumpkin seeds, sunflower seeds and linseeds. Oily fish eaten daily during an outbreak, and three times weekly the rest of the time, is also highly effective. At the same time, keep saturated fats to a minimum so they don't compete with the beneficial effects of the omega-3-rich oils. Flax oil is of benefit, too, and can easily be added into the diet on foods or in shakes. A good proportion of eczema sufferers, along with other atopic allergics, have a faulty enzyme mechanism for converting the essential fat LA into GLA, and these oils provide GLA directly without the need to convert it. Taking a supplement with B-vitamins (for the B6) alongside the evening primrose oil helps its use as well. For different reasons, it also helps skin repair if you pierce a capsule of vitamin E and rub into the affected area daily. If you have trouble encouraging children to take the beneficial oils, pierce a couple of 500 mg capsules of evening primrose, starflower or black-currant oil, and rub them daily into the soft skin inside the arms and the thighs where they are easily absorbed – you can also apply them to the affected areas. If this dose is not effective double it, and for adults take a slightly higher dose.

I have emphasised the necessity of adding foods into the diet for eczema because studies show that nutritional deficiencies rather than food sensitivities or allergies are more common in adults with this condition. Children, however, seem to benefit more from dietary exclusions and, looking at the available trials, I would estimate that about 50 per cent of children with eczema are affected by food sensitivities, the most common being dairy, eggs, soya, citrus fruit, wheat, chocolate, peanuts and potatoes. Coffee also may be a no-no (for adults obviously – I hope!) and trials have shown that atopic eczema in heavy coffee drinkers (ten cups a day) was resolved or improved considerably when coffee drinking was drastically reduced or cut out altogether.

If you have a skin condition you usually also need to pay attention to bowel health. If you go to the loo less than once a day, have irritable bowel syndrome (IBS) or any other digestive condition, address this as a priority. The most important factors to consider are fibre levels in your diet and beneficial bacteria supplementation. Eating a diet rich in vegetables, fruit, pulses and whole grains helps (although make sure you are not sensitive to any of the grains). Adding one or two teaspoons of psyllium husks is the easiest way of improving bowel health, whether you tend towards constipation or loose stools. For information about beneficial bacteria see **Allergic Colitis**, page 79.

The herbs yellow dock (1 teaspoon of the liquid extract in water) and burdock root (3 x 500 mg capsules 2–3 times daily with meals) are also standbys for dealing with eczema. Some products are made with combinations of these herbs and also contain sarsaparilla to help reduce itching.

Many people obtain considerable relief from eczema by visiting a specialist in Chinese herbal medicine and taking the, not very pleasant tasting, herbal brews prescribed. While this can be effective for a few months, it is not uncommon for the eczema to recur more strongly at a later date. Suspicion has fallen on the fact that some herbal compounds are found to contain steroids. If you want to investigate this option, make sure that you see a qualified herbal therapist listed in one of the registers.

For short-term, but effective, relief when experiencing an outbreak, run yourself a soothing bath laced with a handful of chamomile (or use 3/4 teabags) or with 1 cup of oats. Finally, a poultice of grated potato or grated cucumber applied to the affected area seems to help considerably.

HAY FEVER

Just as most people are beginning to enjoy longer, brighter days of spring, a significant minority, about 15–20 per cent, dread the onset of symptoms of hay fever – itchy, watering eyes, streaming or blocked noses, tight throats, wheezing and sneezing and even thumping heads. The sensitivity to pollens that many people suffer, can also be made worse by the rising pollution levels that often accompany warmer temperatures inside cities. You might think that living in the country would automatically make the risk of hay fever worse because of exposure to crops, but studies show that urban living increases the chance of susceptibility. This may be because of increased exposure to other factors, such as house dust mites and pollution, which lead to a compound effect.

Hay fever, which was much rarer only a hundred years ago, is triggered by an over-sensitivity to pollens, but may be made worse by pollution, diet and lifestyle. The main advice is usually to avoid the pollens and take antihistamines. Avoiding foods that come from the same family as the pollens to which the person is sensitive can also reduce the severity of symptoms, or eliminate them altogether. I have seen many cases of hay fever resolved by changes to diet which support the immune system and act as natural antihistamines, and eliminating foods that worsen the condition.

Tree pollen sensitivities usually occur earlier in the year than grass pollen sensitivities and are over by the end of May. Grass pollen sensitivities can happen over a much wider time period during the spring and summer and are responsible for about 90 per cent of cases. The milder winters we are experiencing are leading to a longer hay fever season. Not so long ago, little pollen was seen before April, but now tree pollens are around from March. Each decade since 1970 has seen the season beginning five days earlier.

Timing of symptoms	What you may be allergic to
March–May	alder, hazel and willow
April–May	birch, oak and pine
May–June	oil seed rape
June–August	grass pollen, weed and nettle
August–October	moulds, fungal spores and weeds

If tree pollen sensitivity is your problem, try avoiding hazelnuts, celery, carrots, swede, parsnip and potato during the season in which you are normally sensitive, to see if it makes a difference, since these often cross react. During the rest of the year you may well find that you can tolerate them, though simply peeling, scrubbing or chopping these vegetables during the sensitive season can make symptoms worse for some people.

Grass and pollen sensitivities are much more widespread

and, as a result, the types of foods that can make symptoms worse are more numerous:

● Milk (cow's, goat's and sheep's) and all milk products, including cheese. Ruminants feed on grass, and therefore dairy products can contain grass allergens.

● Many cereals are also members of the grass family, including wheat, barley, rye and oats (though oats are the least likely to cause problems).

● There can be cross-reactions with other allergens, so other foods that may be worth avoiding to see if it makes a difference include: all beans (including soya), lentils, peas, peanuts, tapioca and senna (in medications).

Of course, a diet that excludes these foods can end up being a little restrictive and ideas for foods to use as alternatives are covered in the **Appendices**, page 151.

In order to gain the most benefit, you need to begin your dietary measures a month or two before the likely onset of symptoms, not halfway through the allergy season. If you are unlucky enough to have symptoms related to both tree and grass pollens, you may have to start with the tree pollen exclusion diet as soon as your symptoms start (or preferably before), and then start avoiding the foods related to the grass pollen sensitivities at the beginning of April.

If avoiding these foods helps you, you can challenge your symptoms by reintroducing each of the foods separately, in a methodical way. You may find that you only need to avoid one or two of the foods and not the whole lot. Best results are achieved by cutting them all out in one go rather than cutting them out one by one, as a sensitivity to one can mask the results of cutting out another food.

Sugar is often implicated in hay fever symptoms and avoiding table sugar and sugary foods may help enormously. This is unlikely to be because the sugar cane is in the same botanical family as grasses (as is the case with cereals), but is probably because excess sugar in the diet has the effect of suppressing the immune system.

Vitamin C, 1–3 g daily (taken in divided doses), can act as a natural antihistamine and benefits some people – experiment with this for at least four weeks to see if it helps you. The effect of vitamin C may also be enhanced by taking 500 mg of quercitin, another antihistamine antioxidant, alongside it, two or three times daily. Another possible source of relief is to take a 450 mg capsule of nettle leaf two or three times daily, or an equivalent of nettle leaf tincture (2–4 ml three times daily). Vitamin A, 6,000 ius, 1,800 mcg daily, can help reduce inflammation of the mucus membranes.

Useful homeopathic remedies include pulsatilla, euphrasia, siliceaarsen alb and can be of benefit for children, as tablets just dissolve under the tongue. Nelsons make a hay fever remedy called Pollenna (containing allium, cepa, euphrasia, sabidilla) which can be particularly effective.

Herbs such as liquorice, horseradish and garlic ease irritation though do not take liquorice if you are taking steroids. Other herbal remedies must only be tried with the help of a qualified herbal practitioner, as they can lead to adverse reactions if not used carefully. Herbs which can cause symptoms of hay fever are sometimes used as remedies, such as goldenrod, ragweed, common plaintain, eyebright and elder. Ephedra sinica (Ma huang) is also used, and synthetic ephedrine is the basis of familiar over-the-counter hay fever remedies. There are safety concerns about herbal ephedra (which is only available by prescription or from a qualified herbal practitioner) and it may not be advised.

A drop of eucalyptus, chamomile or lavender aromatherapy oil can be sprinkled on to a handkerchief and sniffed for relief, added to a basin of hot water and inhaled, or added to baths or vaporised at night to aid sleep. Natural eye soothers can include cucumber slices rubbed over the eyes, rosewater-steeped cotton pads and used teabags placed over the eyes for five minutes.

Another simple trick to experiment with is to smooth a non-irritating cream such as Vaseline inside your nose. This literally acts as a barrier that traps the pollen in your lower nostrils and prevents it from setting up an allergic reaction.

Small children under the age of two are not often affected by hay fever and it usually develops around the age of nine to 11. It is more common in allergic, atopic, families, though you can reduce the risk of your child developing it by breast-feeding for the first six months, which builds up the baby's immune resistance. It is also helpful to keep your child away from potentially allergenic foods, such as cow's milk, gluten grains and eggs for their first year.

HEADACHES AND MIGRAINES

Headaches can take many different forms and occur with varying degrees of severity. Serious headaches can last for days or even weeks at a time and, contary to the old joke, men are more prone to them than women. Migraines, on the other hand, are twice as common in women than men and usually last for one or two days at a time, with varying rates of recurrence. They are often brought on by bright lights, lack of sleep, stress and dietary factors.

Migraines are not just more serious headaches – they are a different problem altogether. They are related to the clumping of red blood platelets in the brain's blood supply, which release a brain chemical called serotonin. This leads to a clamping down of the blood vessels, which in the first phase of a migraine is characterised by visual disturbances, dizziness, an increase in hunger and changed sensations on one side of the face. As the reduced blood supply to the brain is detected, there is a reflex reaction which causes a swing in the other direction and the blood vessels over-dilate. The surge of circulation leads to the stage of migraine characterised by thumping and throbbing.

Everyone's migraine is different and symptoms can include head pain (often one-sided), nausea and vomiting, seeing bright lights and visual disturbances. It has been suggested that the distorted faces seen in the work of Picasso owe something to the visual disturbances he suffered during migraine attacks. Migraine attacks in children differ to those of adults, being of shorter duration and often accompanied by stomach aches.

If you have previously been headache- or migraine-free, and are experiencing a sudden onset, you should always be examined by your doctor to ensure that there are not more serious underlying conditions.

Nutritional factors play a significant part for many people with recurrent headaches and migraines, but other factors can be important as well. Tension and stress often contribute to headaches and migraines, particularly when they lead to muscle tensions around the neck, shoulders and back. It is always worth consulting an osteopath, chiropractor or similar to ascertain if there are any physical reasons for the problem, such as a pinched nerve. Many people find that massage, shiatsu, acupuncture or cranial-osteopathy can help to relieve muscle tension, as can posture realignment using disciplines such as the Alexander technique or Pilates.

How to beat headaches

It is wise to concentrate on foods that give consistent energy levels instead of subjecting yourself to the peaks and troughs of blood sugar swings. Eating a diet consisting predominantly of beans, lentils, whole grains, fruit and vegetables can help.

Caffeine is a frequent source of headaches, particularly if you go without for a while. It is common to experience week-end headaches as caffeine intake drops to lower levels than those normal at work during the week. Simply not drinking caffeine overnight can be enough to induce a morning headache which only lifts when you take your first sip of coffee. This leads to the mistaken conclusion that caffeine resolves headache problems, whereas what really happens is that withdrawal symptoms are being knocked on the head with your first gulp of caffeine. Caffeine is put in headache medication not because it solves headaches, but because it makes you more responsive to the painkiller compounds. Drinking as little as one or two cups a day can be enough to cause a headache when you don't get your fix. Decaffeinated coffee or tea is the answer for some people, although others remain sensitive to the caffeine-like compounds – theophylline and theobromine – that remain. Some people find it easier to wean themselves off slowly to avoid rebound headaches, others just accept that the best way is to go cold turkey, suffer the headaches for a couple of days or more, and then experience the clarity that comes with a headache-free existence.

I have seen many people's long-term problems with headaches resolve completely, or at least improve significantly, after avoiding the two things upon which so much blame seems to be laid – wheat and dairy-based foods. Again it is a matter of trial and error, but this is worth trying because it seems to work so well, so often. See **Appendices**, pages 152-56, for alternative foods.

MSG (monosodium glutamate), which is used extensively as a food preservative and flavouring, and is particularly common in Chinese food, may also lead to headaches. The term Chinese

Restaurant Syndrome was coined to describe the effects, which include headaches with perspiration and a difficulty catching breath, that eating MSG has on some people.

Painkiller abuse is another fairly common reason for headaches. A vicious circle is created when attempts to subdue the headache with painkillers leads to an increase in the number and frequency with which they are taken. Painkillers need to be processed in the liver, and an overload of the capability of the liver to function means that toxins then trigger the headaches. Even children have been found to suffer for this reason. In one clinic, children between the ages of 6–16 stopped taking analgesics, which resulted in the clearing of headaches in two-thirds of them. Excess alcohol (which can mean a comparatively small amount if the person is sensitive) can also perpetuate headaches for the same reason – it overloads the liver.

Headaches are also commonly brought on by a susceptibility to chemicals and perfumes. Avoiding the source, for example dry-cleaning fluids, car exhausts and scented products, is advisable, but the condition may be a warning that your liver needs detoxification (see *The Detox Manual* in this series of books).

Magnesium is probably one of the most effective remedies for headache sufferers, and is a good muscle relaxant. A dose of 400–600 mg needs to be taken daily for at least a month to restore low magnesium levels in the body, this can then be reduced to 250–300 mg. This works best when taken alongside a 50 mg B-complex.

Ginger is an age-old remedy for headaches that really works, and keeping a jar of crystallised ginger handy for when you feel a headache coming on is a delicious way to see it off. For the more puritanical, you can chew on a piece of ginger root or drink ginger tea. Other beneficial teas (which are available as teabags) include lime flower, scullcap and lemon verbena.

A couple of drops (in total) of lavender and/or peppermint aromatherapy oil applied to the temples can be very effective in banishing a headache. Lavender is calming and a natural analgesic, while peppermint helps to relax the muscles around the head.

How to beat migraines

Whatever you do, do not skip meals, and make sure you eat at regular times, as migraines can be brought on by simply missing out on one meal. It is also a good idea to keep your blood sugar level constant by snacking on wholesome (not sugary) snacks in between meals. And so you don't get caught out, keep health bars, oatcakes or similar in your bag or car for emergencies. Make sure, too, that you eat a little before exercising, as it can bring blood sugar levels down and trigger an attack. It is also wise to have a light snack just before going to bed to take you through the night.

Migraine sufferers are usually aware of the potential of 'the five Cs' – chocolate, cheese, claret (i.e. wine), coffee and citrus fruit – to cause problems. Up to 25 per cent of migraines seem to be related to food and drink, and the most common culprits are alcohol, chocolate, cheese and other dairy foods and citrus fruit, which are rich sources of vasoactive amines which trigger the blood vessels in the brain.

Rather than having an allergy to certain foods, up to 25 per cent of migraine sufferers are deficient in an important enzyme, PST (phenolsulphotransferase), which normally inactivates certain compounds – proteins called amines. Low levels of PST mean that amine levels rise, stimulating the platelets to clump together, which in turn releases serotonin. Common sources of these unhelpful amine compounds are tyramine-rich blue and mature cheeses (but not cream or cottage cheese) and red wine (Chianti, in particular, can be very tyramine-rich). Red wine is also a rich source of phenolic flavonoid compounds, as is chocolate. These flavonoids give them their colour, but can also inactivate PST. Alcohol is also a vasodilator (which means it dilates blood vessels). Other tyramine-rich foods are Marmite, Horlicks, liver, sausages, broad beans and pickled herrings. Fruit and vegetables develop increased tyramine concentrations when they become overripe, thus foods such as overripe avocados and canned figs can be culprits. Phenylethylamine, another amine compound, is also found in chocolate, and the darker the chocolate the more it contains. Other amines are histamine, found in wine, beer, cheese, salami and pickled foods (see **Appendices**, page 171), and octopamine and synephrine, found in oranges and other citrus fruit, their juices and marmalade.

Other foods linked to migraines are caffeinated drinks, nuts, fried and fatty foods, and pork, which is implicated more often than other meats. Nitrates and nitrites, which are used in cured meats such as bacon, salami and frankfurters, can trigger unpleasant similar effects to those described previously, with an initial constriction of blood vessels in the brain, followed by dilation of the blood vessels. Nitrates are also found in smaller quantities in foods such as beetroot, celery, lettuce, radishes, rhubarb and spinach.

Aspartame is an artificial sweetener used in many soft drinks, yoghurts and other manufactured, sweet-tasting foods, and as a sugar substitute. It is made from two amino acids, phenylalanine and aspartic acid. In one study, more than one in ten people thought their migraines were brought on by this sweetener.

Not all of the potential culprit foods cause problems for all people all of the time. The only way to ascertain if any might be involved for you is to keep a meticulous food diary while eating normally, or to go on a diet that initially excludes the triggers and then reintroduces them.

The omega-3 fats found in oily fish, when eaten regularly,

can reduce the frequency and intensity of attacks significantly, as they reduce the clumping of red blood cells.

St John's wort can be useful for some migraine sufferers as it has the effect of balancing four neurotransmitters (nerve chemicals) in the brain. It is most likely to be effective when taken alongside another complementary herbs such as valerian or kava kava. Do not, however, take St John's wort alongside migraine medication as it can interact with the drug by clearing it more quickly through the liver.

Bowel health is always of paramount importance when dealing with migraines, or headaches for that matter, so please refer back to the information given in **Strategies For Allergies**, page 39.

As with headaches, supplementing the mineral magnesium at around 400–600 mg daily for a month, and then cutting back to 250–300 mg, can be a remarkably effective way of avoiding migraine attacks. It is estimated that magnesium deficiency is linked to 50 per cent of migraine problems. Good sources of magnesium in the diet include green leafy vegetables, fresh seeds, fresh nuts, dried fruit, seafood, wholegrains, brewer's yeast and soya beans. There has also been research done that shows that high doses of riboflavin (vitamin B2), well in excess of the amount found in most supplements, has a marked effect on reducing the frequency of migraines, with the participants in the trial suffering 37 per cent fewer migraines after taking the B2 for two months than those taking placebos. The study used 400 mg daily, as against the upper end of most high dose supplements which give 50–100 mg. It is always advisable to take a high dose single B-vitamin, such as taking this amount of B2, alongside a B-complex giving around 50 mg of all the other B-vitamins. As vitamin B2 is water soluble this amount should not pose any toxicity problems.

The herb considered most effective for migraine, when

taken regularly, is feverfew, and scientific trials back this up. The active agent in feverfew is parthenolide, which reduces the platelet-clumping action that triggers migraine. It can be taken as a tea (made with feverfew infusion), as a tincture in the morning (50 drops) or by adding one or two leaves to salads or sandwiches (but do not eat more than this). Feverfew grows easily in the garden or in a pot on the window-sill, which means you can always have a fresh supply of leaves, though make sure you have the right variety, *Tanacetum parthenium*. It can take a month of taking feverfew daily for the effects to be noticed, so be patient. Do not take feverfew if you are taking blood-thinning medication such as Warfarin.

Butterbur root (*Petasites hybridus*) is another herb which is proving useful and which has been used in Germany for a while. As with feverfew it is most useful when used to stave off migraines, by taking it on a regular basis. The dose is a 50 mg capsule twice daily.

Chamomile tea is also soothing – make a strong brew, steeping for four or five minutes, and drink up to five cups daily.

Migraines are twice as likely around the first couple of days of menstruation and least likely around ovulation time. For women who find that migraines are triggered around the time of their period, the herb chaste berry (*Agnus castus* or *Vitex agnus castus*) can bring relief after it has been taken for two or three months, as it has the effect of balancing hormones that can trigger attacks when they are out of synch. Conversely, the oral contraceptive pill and HRT can trigger migraines in some women.

INSECT STINGS/BITES

It is reasonably common to be allergic to insect bites and stings and, though an anaphylactic reaction is rare, they can lead to very uncomfortable and itchy weals that take a considerable time to heal. This can be particularly irritating in the summer, when you are likely to be confronted with more insects than you would like. The spring is therefore a good time to focus on lowering histamine levels by following the advice given in **Reducing Your Histamine Reaction**, page 63.

Mosquitoes dislike the taste of B vitamins on the skin, so if you are taking a high dose B-complex of 100 mg daily this can help to repel them. Certain essential oils also act as insect repellents, including mint, eucalyptus, citrus, citronella and clove oil, and burning them, particularly in a bedroom at night, can be very effective. You can also massage an insect repellant oil on to your skin. Mix five drops of cedarwood and ten drops of lavender oil into 10 ml of a base oil, such as almond oil, then smooth this on to exposed areas. Mosi-guard is a product which uses all natural ingredients, lemon and eucalyptus oils, and is effective. If you get stung by a wasp, vinegar dabbed on the area will help, and if it is a bee sting then bicarbonate will help. Neither of these are effective if you have a bad allergy however.

OTITIS MEDIA (GLUE EAR)

This condition, found in children, is a build-up of sticky fluid in the middle ear, and is usually the result of repeated infections or allergy. Glue ear is on the increase and 40 per cent of children under the age of six experience this problem. It is often diagnosed because a child seems to be slightly deaf; if allowed to go undetected it can cause them to be labelled inattentive. The usual treatment, in the case of infection, is antibiotics, but if the situation does not improve then grommets are inserted into the ear canal under general anaesthetic. This is an unpleasant procedure which can usually be avoided. While antibiotics may be necessary to clear up an infection crisis (which in children is vital because inner ear infections can lead to deafness) improving immune health and reducing susceptibility due to food sensitivities can prevent infection in the first place (see **Strategies For Allergies**, page 39). Antibiotics are a double-edged sword and children who are given several courses often end up being more susceptible to glue ear.

The main food culprits linked to otitis media are dairy produce, sugar and wheat. It is extremely common to find that children who suffer from glue ear have a diet which involves a lot of milk, as well as the other two foods. Any child with glue ear needs to avoid milk and cheese totally. If this does not produce results, suspect other foods. Your child's hearing should always be checked a few weeks after an ear infection.

Sometimes help comes in the most unexpected forms – in this case chewing gum! You may not like the idea of your child chewing like a cow, but there may be good reasons to do so. Research has shown that chewing sugar-free gum sweetened with xylitol five times a day for five minutes each time reduces the episodes of glue ear by 45 per cent. Xylitol is a type of sugar that does not affect dental health adversely, and it is not a chemically-derived synthetic sweetener. The reason it works is because the xylitol prevents troublesome bacteria from sticking to the mucus lining of the naso-pharyngeal area. Children as young as one and three quarters were successfully able to chew the gum in the trials, but I would not advise this because of the risk of choking. Children should always be supervised while chewing gum.

PSORIASIS

Psoriasis is a chronic scaling disease of the skin. Normally, the outer layer of dead skin cells are shed and replaced at a consistent rate, but in psoriasis they are not shed fast enough to keep up with the vastly increased production of new cells underneath. This leads to the characteristically high levels of keratinocytes (surface skin cells) and scaling. If the scales are removed pin-point bleeding occurs.

Around 2 per cent of Western populations, i.e. around a million people in the UK, have some form of psoriasis and it usually first manifests itself between the ages of ten and 30, though it can occur at any time, even in babies. There are several types of psoriasis, the most common being the plaque-type, which mainly affects the legs, arms and buttocks. Guttate psoriasis in children often starts after a throat infection and does not necessarily lead to plaque type psoriasis in adulthood. Erythrodermic, or pustular, psoriasis is severe and requires medical supervision as secondary infections are a possible complication.

Three quarters of sufferers have a particular gene which seems to be linked to the disease, and a third of them have a family history of the disease, especially if it develops early. Psoriasis is sometimes described as a genetic time bomb waiting to explode when the conditions are right. While psoriasis is generally considered incurable, there is no doubt that careful management can put many cases into long-term remission.

The effect of hormones on the condition can be unpredictable. Eight out of ten female psoriasis sufferers find that pregnancy improves the condition, suggesting that the hormones of pregnancy have a beneficial effect. However, some women find that symptoms appear for the first time after they have their first baby, which suggests to me that nutritional imbalances or deficiencies might be exacerbated by pregnancy, stress or tiredness in susceptible people. A change in circumstances is the trigger for many conditions and it has been observed that Australian Aboriginal people, for example, do not suffer from psoriasis when living in the bush and following a traditional lifestyle, but develop it when they move to the city.

Psoriasis is often treated with ultraviolet light which can be effective for mild to moderate psoriasis, though some find that exposure worsens their condition. Vitamin D is made in the skin on exposure to ultraviolet light, and fish oils, which are an effective treatment for psoriasis, are high in this vitamin. Vitamin D derivatives (calcipotriol and tacalcitol) in ointment are available on prescription and are used to reduce plaque psoriasis. Emollient creams are also applied which soften and soothe the skin, and these sometimes contain antipuritics to reduce itching. Coal tar extract is messy and smells unpleasant, but is part of the standard treatment package.

The nutritional management of psoriasis begins quite definitely with essential fatty acids. The skin of people with psoriasis contains large amounts of free-arachadonic acid (AA), which is easily converted to lipoxygenase substances that are believed to play an important role in worsening the condition. The omega-3 fats found in fish oils and flax oil are particularly beneficial, and eating a large portion (200 g) of oily fish daily can make a great difference. Supplementing with fish oils can also improve the situation, but the amount needed to make a significant difference, 5 g or more, can cause unpleasant 'repeating'. It is much more agreeable, and extremely effective, to take 1 or 2 tablespoons of cold pressed flax oil daily, more if you are experiencing a flare-up, and less for general management. Flax oil contains a good balance of omega-3 and omega-6 fatty acids, which lead to a good ratio of PGE1 and PGE3 and can reduce inflammation and itching. If you find taking flax oil in liquid form difficult, try capsules instead – 1-2 g three times daily with food. You can also take supplements which blend the flax oil with pumpkin and borage seed oil.

At the same time as dramatically increasing your essential fatty acid intake, cut back on animal fat (and therefore meat, cheese, butter, etc), since its consumption leads to PGE2 production, which actively counteracts the benefits of the PGE1 and PGE3. Oily fish, white fish and some game meats (which have a better fat profile than other red meats) are better options.

For cases of psoriasis that are not too extensive, try, as an alternative to cortisone creams, ointments which contain soothing chamomile, comfrey, which aids skin healing, and liquorice, which has a cortisone-like effect (see **Resources**, page 185). One study came to the conclusion that liquorice-based cream was more effective than cortisone cream with 93 per cent of the study group reporting benefits from using this cream against 83 per cent in the group using cortisone cream.

It is worth investigating food sensitivities, though they have a less clear link with psoriasis than with other conditions. Dairy products can cause problems, as can oranges and other citrus fruits. If eating citrus fruit has a negative effect, you may also need to avoid vitamin C supplements. While vitamin C is generally superb for skin healing, some supplements may aggravate this condition though the non-acidic forms are best (magnesium ascorbate, calcium ascorbate, sodium ascorbate and Ester-C). Good food sources of vitamin C which can be increased in the diet are kiwi fruit, strawberries, other berries, broccoli and cabbage. Foods which are sources of polyamines can also be involved with psoriasis, which means experimenting with the usual cast of suspects: alcohol, dairy produce, meats and chocolate. Sugar and gluten grains (wheat, barley, rye and oats) are other possible suspects. If the condition persists sufficiently for you to need to investigate this list it is important to make sure your diet is not too restricted, so follow the elimination diet given in **Appendices**, page 148. It may also be worth considering having an ELISA blood test (see **Allergy Tests**, page 178) to work out which food sensitivities, if any, play a part in the condition.

In many cases, drinking too much alcohol or smoking can exacerbate the disease, particularly for those with pustular psoriasis, and it is best to avoid these twin aggravators.

Coleus forskohlii is an effective Ayurvedic (Indian) herbal treatment for psoriasis since it increases levels of the chemical cAMP (cyclic-AMP), which is involved in cell manufacture. Excessive proliferation of cells is slowed by higher levels of cAMP. Buy a standardised supplement containing 18 per cent of the active compound forskolin and try a dose of 50 mg three times a day. Milk thistle is a herb normally given for liver health, which is a factor in psoriasis, but it also has the effect of reducing excess cellular proliferation. Take two 100 mg capsules two or three times daily, preferably between meals. Another useful herb is *Berberis aquifolium* (Oregon grape) which, as the common name suggests, comes from North America. You can buy a fluid extract and take a third of a teaspoon three times a day. It may take some time to take effect, but persevere as it is effective.

SINUSITIS AND ALLERGIC RHINITIS

Sinusitis is an inflammation of the membranes lining the sinuses, often due to infection, but also to allergy. The sinuses are cavities in the skull found in the forehead and either side of the nose. When they become blocked, the build up of pressure can be exceedingly uncomfortable. It is not unusual for infected sinuses to be mistaken for toothache, as the pain radiates downwards.

Allergies that most commonly trigger sinusitis include hay fever and sensitivity to animal dander. These are also triggers for rhinitis, a similar problem affecting the membranes lining the nose, including the back of the nose, which lead down to the throat. Common symptoms are a stuffed up sensation, a dripping nose and drip at the back of the nose into the throat, called post-nasal drip. The word catarrh has its root in the Greek *kata* (down) and *rhein* (to flow), which describes its course down the back of the throat rather acurately!

Cat allergies are more common than allergies to dogs, possibly because cats spend more time cleaning themselves and their saliva attaches to their dander. Between 5 and 10 per cent of people are thought to be allergic to cats to some degree. Interestingly, around two thirds of dark haired cats cause problems for sufferers, but only a quarter of light haired ones. People who keep cats in their bedroom, as opposed to the rest of the house, are more likely to suffer a cat allergy. Before you hastily re-house your family pet, with all the attendant problems of explaining this to the children, it is worth investigating food sensitivities, since you may find that dealing with these raises your tolerance to a level whereby you can keep your little friend in the house. Homeopathic desensitisation can also be quite effective in these cases, and for this you need to consult a medically qualified homeopath.

All the usual food sensitivities are capable of worsening both of these conditions, in particular sensitivity to dairy products, which encourage mucus production in the nasal and sinus area, and to gluten grains, particularly wheat. As with most allergy problems, any food could be involved.

Foods which are high in antioxidants can help to reduce the inflammation of the nasal membranes, as well as provide the building blocks for healthy mucus membranes. Of most use are highly coloured fruit and vegetables, such as carrots, for their beta-carotene, blackcurrants and other berries, for their proanthocyanidins, and lemon and orange juice (as long as you do not react to citrus fruit), for their vitamin C content. Garlic has powerful antibacterial properties and clears the nose wonderfully if crushed raw into a salad or mixed with olive oil and spread on bread (again, as long as you do not have a problem with wheat!). Oily fish are also marvellous for maintaining the healthy functioning of the mucus membranes. You may find, too, that the bee product propolis is helpful if you habitually suffer from sinusitis and rhinitis.

Nettle supplements have been shown to reduce the symptoms of allergic rhinitis or, if you are feeling energetic, you can make your own tea or nettle soup. Horseradish and ginger herbal tinctures can also help to ease breathing and reduce nasal congestion.

Steam inhalation is very effective at loosening the mucus in the nasal and face cavities, and some herbal infusions added to the water can help – experiment with eucalyptus, chamomile, thyme, rosemary, mint or tea tree.

URTICARIA (NETTLE RASH)

Urticaria, otherwise known as nettle rash, and hives are the same thing, and are characterised by a collection of red, raised, itchy weals which may also have patches of white scattered amongst them. Food allergy (the classic IgE type) is most often the cause and antihistamines can bring relief in some cases. Sometimes the culprit is easy to recognise if it is an infrequently eaten food, and typically protein foods such as fish or shellfish will often be the source of the problem. The only answer is to avoid the offending food.

Chronic urticaria is defined as wealing and/or angioedema (a swelling of the tissues usually of the face, eyes, lips and tongue) occurring at least twice a week and lasting for longer than six weeks. The condition is often regarded as idiopathic (with no known cause) and specific causes are only identified in 10–20 per cent of cases. Because of this, it is notoriously difficult to treat. Links which are often suggested include infections, drug reactions, pseudoallergic reactions to food additives and IgE allergic reactions, though the relevance of these is inconsistent, and at best can be applied to the individual. Pseudoallergy refers to a reaction that cannot be confirmed with an IgE test.

In an interesting paper reporting a well conducted trial using 64 people with urticaria, remarkably effective results were obtained using a pseudoallergen-free diet. This diet excluded all sources of common chemical allergens, including preservatives, food colours and even many naturally occurring compounds found in fruit and some vegetables. The trials took place in the controlled environment of a hospital and, over a two-week period, three quarters of the people found that their symptoms either totally ceased or were greatly reduced and, on a follow up six months later, half of the people continued to show complete remission and all but one of the remainder had lasting improvements. All the patients were given the same diet. For the first three days only freshly cooked, unsulphited potatoes, polished rice, water and salt were allowed. After this a less restricted diet was allowed, which was free of all artificial additives and the compounds called salicylates found in fruit, spices and vegetables. For the full list of foods both allowed and forbidden see **Appendices**, page 135.

A herb that can be useful for urticaria, and also strawberry and shellfish allergies, is nettle leaf, which you can take as capsules, two or three times daily. Another possible treatment is acupuncture, which has been shown to be effective for treating many cases of urticaria.

CHAPTER NINE

Children and Allergies

As already mentioned, the incidence of allergies in children has increased astoundingly in the last few decades, and in every classroom there is likely to be a list of foods that some children must avoid, plus several inhalers, yet only 50 years ago young asthmatics and children with other allergies were a comparative rarity.

It is heart-rending to see a child who is covered from head to toe in itchy eczema or who is gasping for breath with asthma, and this makes it all the more satisfying to discover effective treatments for these, and similar, conditions. Children are particularly rewarding to work with, because they respond so well to the effects of improved diet on their health; they also respond much more quickly than adults.

As children get older, and particularly when they are exposed to peer group pressure at school, they often form strong opinions about what they want to eat. It is all too easy for the harassed parent to give in to demands for less nutritious foods. But when it comes to foods to which they have adverse reactions, most children are fairly sensible. If they are aware that they need to avoid peanuts or milk, for instance, they will usually do so, and they often remember more readily than their parents which foods contain the forbidden ingredients. Reinforcement of this awareness is, of course, much easier if they have a strong allergic reaction to a food, than if the reaction is delayed or obscure.

Having attractive substitutes for foods they enjoy is an important part of the equation. If they can't have a particular type of biscuit or cake, then it is made much easier for them if they are offered an appealing option. Not many children want to munch on an apple while their friends are digging into a slice of cake, but they may well welcome a piece of flapjack.

Inevitably, numerous obstacles get in the way of investigating a food sensitivity in a child – the school canteen, birthday parties, peer pressure from other children. You will need to approach the problem in two stages – the investigative stage and the maintenance stage. In the first instance, you really need to have a clear two or three weeks to find out what might be affecting your child. Pick a time when you are likely to have a clear run and will be able to avoid being sidetracked. Find pursuits for your child that will avoid contact with too much temptation. Make sure that the whole family is being supportive and eating the same way. Once you are through that stage, it is a question of applying what you, and your child, have learned. This may be more tricky, and you may have to accept that the regime will go off the rails occasionally, perhaps at awkward times. For the most part, if you plan ahead, create a new set of habits and regimes, talk to the child's school and invest some time, if necessary, in preparing packed lunches, your child's health will probably improve dramatically. If there is any resistance to your programme, a dramatic improvement in symptoms is usually all that is needed to turn doubters and cynics into converts!

It is awkward, but not impossible, to wean children off a food to which they are attached, if you need to find out whether it is involved in their allergic condition. If they have been drinking milk or eating bread for four or five years, and you suddenly announce that they can't have their favourite night-time tipple of warm milk or their favourite cereal for breakfast, it is likely to cause a problem. Nevertheless, children, from the age of two upwards, are quite able to join in the whole exercise and it is best to sit them down and talk about what you are planning to do, and why, and in this way they can understand what is going on. Make a project of the exercise and include them in the planning. The only groups of children for whom this approach might not work are those with ADHD (Attention Deficit Hyperactivity Disorder) or autism, though this does not mean that you should not aim to make them understand. (There has, in recent years, been a lot of good work done on autism and food sensitivities, usually involving wheat, dairy and some fruit, and a number of autistic children have responded very well with improved cognitive skills.) It is important not to make a big issue out of food and eating, otherwise the whole exercise can become an unpleasant tug of wills. Be firm and kind, but don't get emotional, otherwise it is almost certain to rebound badly.

Delicious alternative choices

- buckwheat flour pancakes with a little maple syrup instead of toast and jam
- banana-sweetened muffins instead of sugary options
- calcium-enriched rice milk in a fruit smoothie instead of milk
- oatcakes topped with strawberries mashed with honey instead of jam sandwiches
- soya yoghurt instead of milk-laced desserts
- home-made mango, gooseberry or rhubarb fool instead of shop-bought mousse
- dairy-free ice cream
- pastas made from grains other than wheat
- fructose or FOS (fructo-oligo-saccharides), in great moderation, instead of sugar

With any change in routine it is as well to be organised. Before D-day (diet day) gather a supply of substitutes in the food cupboard, refrigerator or freezer. Ideally, experiment by giving these substitutes to your children in advance to make sure they like them. If at first you don't succeed, don't give up but try the same choices on a different day, or alter the recipe. You may find it easier to ease into an elimination diet by slowly reducing the offending food and replacing it with alternatives. The problem with this approach, however, is that you will prolong the time it takes to find out if the food being eliminated is really causing a problem. From the point at which you eliminate the food totally you need to allow a clear two or three weeks before attempting to reintroduce the food again.

MEETING CHILDREN'S NUTRITONAL NEEDS

It is particularly important to make sure that your child's nutritional needs are being met, as they are growing and developing and using loads of energy on schoolwork and physical activity. It is not appropriate to restrict whole food groups. If you need to cut out wheat, for instance, you must find other grains with a similar nutritional value to fill the gap. I have witnessed many cases where parents have eliminated a whole host of foods without adding others as substitutes. Often they end up becoming positively paranoid about food and what their child can and cannot have. This is really not the point of the exercise, and is highly undesirable for the child. I usually spend more time adding foods to these children's diets than eliminating them. The temptation is always to say 'we have got somewhere with eliminating this food, so let's go on and try eliminating others' without giving any thought to what foods should be added. I have also seen children who have been dragged from practitioner to practitioner, each of whom diagnosed different 'allergies' who, by the time they got to me, were in danger of suffering from malnutrition.

These children need dense sources of nutrients and calories. In the case of an allergy such as eczema, for example, food allergies may have a significant part to play, but then so do nutritional deficiencies. It is just as important to build the child up with sources of essential fats, from cold pressed oils, seeds, oily fish and evening primrose oil, and to find out about any possible vitamin and mineral deficiencies as it is to check out food elimination diets (see the section on boosting the immune system, pages 45-49).

If your child needs to eliminate foods for a while it can do no harm, and may do a lot of good, particularly if a multivitamin and mineral supplement is taken. Supplements should never, however, be used as an alternative to nutrient-rich foods. It is also possible for some supplements to cause allergy, due to colourings and fillers.

Ascertaining if there really is a need to restrict a child's diet, and then embarking on an elimination programme can be difficult, mainly because of the need for co-operation from the child. But generally, as long as you do not eliminate whole classes of foods, it can be managed perfectly well. The food groups which you need to include in your child's diet, or for that matter in an adult's diet, are:

proteins meat, poultry, fish, eggs, cheese, beans, pulses, nuts, seeds
carbohydrates bread, cereals, pasta, potatoes, crispbreads, cakes, biscuits
fruit and vegetables all fruit and vegetables (though potatoes are carbohydrates)
calcium-rich foods milk, yoghurt, calcium-enriched dairy alternatives (i.e. soya or rice milks), canned fish (sardines,

salmon), green leafy vegetables (cabbage, kale, broccoli, brussels sprouts), nuts, seeds, eggs, dried fruit, wholegrain cereals

fats oily fish, nuts, seeds, oils (flax, olive and other cold pressed oils), avocados, egg yolks, butter, coconut

Children need to be treated cautiously because of the many demands of a growing body, and it is always best to consult your doctor, as well as a nutritional therapist or dietician. Young children should never be put on a rigid exclusion diet without expert help. However, avoiding common foods to which they react, such as cow's milk, eggs, food additives and sugar, can usually be accomplished quite safely, as long as nutritious substitutes are found so you do not leave nutritional holes in the child's diet.

The advice given so far in this book is generally suitable for children, though because supplement and herbal doses have been given for adults, with children it is best to work with a qualified nutritionist or herbalist to ensure what your child takes is safe.

If a child is being breast-fed and is exhibiting signs of possible allergy or sensitivity to food, such as eczema or colic, it is possible they are reacting to foods in the mother's diet which are affecting the breast milk. The most common culprits for this, again, are cow's milk, eggs and wheat, but often also the onion family (including garlic and leeks). It is also common for the mother to be low in essential fats, which manifests itself as symptoms in the breast-fed child.

ASTHMA IN CHILDREN – PRECAUTIONS

With asthma, reintroducing foods can sometimes cause a severe reaction. Because asthma is so prevalent in children, and because real harm can be done by reintroducing foods in the wrong circumstances (principally with brittle asthma), and also because it can be challenging to get a child to change diet, here is a guide as to whether foods should be suspected in the first place:

● If the child's asthma is mild to moderate, and they have no other health problems, there is only a small likelihood that food sensitivities will play a part. In these cases more success is likely to be found by looking at other areas, such as house dust mites and pets. You can certainly experiment with food avoidance, which might yield results, but you may well be disappointed. Enhancing the child's nutritional status, for instance by increasing beneficial fats, is most likely to be helpful.

● If there are other symptoms apart from the asthma, such as digestive complaints, nausea, constipation, diarrhoea, mouth ulcers, headaches, migraines, water retention, aching muscles, glue ear or a vague feeling of being unwell, suspect a food intolerance, and work out which foods need to be eliminated. The most likely culprits are dairy, eggs, wheat, soya and sugar. It is quite safe to experiment, as long as you remember to take care of your child's nutritional needs. See **Appendices**, page 151, for alternative sources of common foods.

● If you note that a particular food, or foods, make asthma attacks worse you can suspect other foods as well because if one intolerance exists it is common for others to occur alongside it. Again, it is quite safe to experiment to try to identify them, as long as you remember to look after your child's nutritional needs.

● In the case of brittle asthma you must be very cautious as this is the most severe kind of asthma. On the plus side, as many as 60 per cent respond to food intolerance investigations. However, considerable caution needs to be exercised, as the risk of a potentially dangerous asthma attack is greater with brittle asthma when foods are reintroduced and tested. In brittle asthma, the reaction to foods that are reintroduced after an avoidance period can be severe, even if they were eaten frequently previously. It is only advisable to test the foods when under close medical supervision, and ideally in hospital. Brittle asthmatics tend to have a lower dietary intake of magnesium and the antioxidant vitamins A, C and E than the recommended nutrient intake, so special attention may need to be paid to increasing their nutritional status. (See pages 87-95 for more general information about asthma.)

DIET AND BEHAVIOUR

One aspect of children's health which is rarely thought of as being linked to diet and allergies is that of behaviour and hyper-activity or ADHD (Attention Deficit Hyperactivity Disorder). The causes of ADHD are not understood, but it is thought that it is a result of a hereditary predisposition combined with environmental factors. There has been fairly convincing evidence in recent years of a link between ADHD and exposure to lead, cigarette smoke, alcohol, chemicals and poor diet while the baby is in the womb. But the link to the child's diet and behaviour remains fairly controversial.

In the 1970s Dr Benjamin Feingold, a medical allergy specialist in California, found that treating children with diet led to a significant improvement in problems with hyperactivity, as well as skin rashes, asthma and other allergic reactions. His work was criticised, however, for not being 'controlled' (in other words not being conducted under laboratory conditions) and as a result was considered just a hypothesis. Nevertheless, many desperate parents who treated their children along the lines he suggested found that their children experienced relief from their behavioural problems. In a 1990 review of diet and behaviour, Dr C. Keith Connors at the University of Pittsburgh said: 'I have to admit that I have changed my mind about the Feingold idea since the 1970s . . . my judgement is that the evidence is strong enough, at least for preschoolers, and especially for those with confirmed allergic symptoms, that one should eliminate a broad range of unnecessary and possibly harmful ingredients from these children's diets.' To bring the story up to date, the Center for Science in the Public Interest, based in Washington DC, has recently conducted a review of 23 controlled studies, and found that 17 of these concluded that some children's behaviour significantly worsened after consumption of artificial colours or some specific foods such as milk or wheat. A trial reported in *The Lancet* concluded that 62 out of 76 overactive children (or 82 per cent) treated with an elimination diet improved, and the behaviour of 21 of these children (more than one-third) became completely normal.

There are four main dietary changes to make with children who have behavioural problems, to evaluate if they work. If your child has been prescribed medication to alleviate the symptoms of ADHD then a trial of six to eight weeks of dietary change may be sufficient to ensure that your child need not go on to the medication, which has side effects, as does any drug. The main changes to experiment with are:

● Avoiding all sources of sugar (see **Appendices**, pages 160-61).
● Assessing whether your child has a problem with particular food sensitivities, particularly to wheat or dairy products (see **Appendices**, pages 152-56).
● Avoiding all artificial food colourings, which have been linked to hyperactivity (see **Appendices**, pages 168-171).

● If the above measures do not work fully, ascertain if your
child has a sensitivity to salicylates in foods (see
Appendices, pages 172-74).

Your child may need some supplements to correct
nutritional deficiencies. Particularly concentrate on essential
fats: fish oils, flax oil and evening primrose oil. Zinc and
magnesium are also usually very important and they can also
help to eliminate unwanted metals which may be affecting
nervous tissue. B-vitamins improve many cases, though in rare
instances the child reacts badly to them. Any supplement plan
should be put together by a trained nutritionist.

There are other possibilities to investigate if the above either
do not work, or do not work fully, but these need professional
support. The child's heavy metal (lead, cadmium, etc) status can
be looked at, thyroid function may need to be checked and a
higher protein diet may be advised. Do not attempt any of these
on your own, instead see a doctor who works with a nutritionist and has an interest in these matters.

GETTING OFF TO THE RIGHT START

It is always easier to start properly at the beginning than to back-
track, particularly as small children are often more susceptible
to problems than adults because of their immature digestive and
immune systems. Weaning children properly can make all the
difference as to whether or not they develop allergies in the first
place.

I frequently see small children of two and three years old
who are in great pain from constipation, but who won't go to the
lavatory until they finally have no choice, and who, as a result,
have anal bleeding and severe pain from passing stools. All this
can, usually, be eliminated in an instant by avoiding cow's milk

and substituting calcium-enriched rice or oat milk in dishes such as desserts, hot chocolate and shakes (soya milk can also be an appropriate alternative, but it elicits allergy problems in a significant number of dairy-allergic children). And the warning signs are always there. On closer questioning, the parents remember that they noticed diarrhoea, colic, nappy rashes or eczema when the baby was weaned, but because milk is considered 'good' for babies they persevered. 'Why weren't we told earlier?' the parents always say.

Breast-fed babies are more likely to be allergy-free babies, and continuing until the baby is at least six months old is a good idea, though a year is better. Foods are best not introduced before four months, and waiting until six months is usually fine (it depends on the baby). When you do introduce foods keep those that are most likely to be allergenic for later, because the baby's digestive tract is immature and may react if exposed too early. And when you stop breast-feeding, introduce a formula milk, not ordinary cow's milk. Even so, a significant number of children react badly to coming off the breast and on to bottle milk, so look out for symptoms such as changed bowel habits, skin eruptions and colic.

For information about weaning babies and the best way to avoid allergies see my book, *What Should I Feed My Baby?*

Part Five

APPENDICES

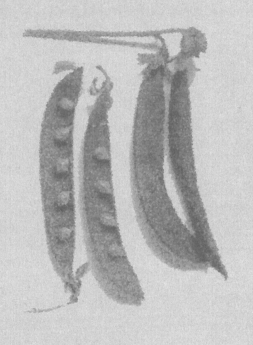

Introduction

The nature of allergies is that they vary greatly from person to person — a reflection of our biochemical individuality. Most people will find that their allergic symptoms improve dramatically, or even clear up, if they follow the advice outlined so far in this book. This consists mainly of improving your intake of essential fats, ensuring that your intake of nutrients beneficial for skin and mucus membrane health is good, supporting your immune health and avoiding the foods to which you might be sensitive.

My intention throughout the book was to keep the advice as simple as possible, because it is so easy to be overwhelmed with information on this topic. However, there are some people who inevitably find they need to educate themselves on the sources of different foods or delve deeper into the problems surrounding their allergies, and the Appendices have been compiled with them in mind. The lists can seem a little complicated and overwhelming, but there is no need to read them all. If you want, you can scan them to get an idea of what they are about, and then forget about them unless you need to use specific lists.

Rotation Plan

Do not attempt a rotation diet unless you really feel that you need to. Rotation diets are, in one sense, quite simple and straightforward, but in terms of fitting them in to a 'normal' life they can be quite awkward. It is probably best to follow a rotation diet only if you have no choice, because you can't get to the bottom of your food intolerance problems. They are suitable for the small minority of people with multiple food allergies and sensitivities. If you find that you are reacting to a large number of foods and you eliminate them all, there is a risk that you can end up with a seriously nutritionally-depleted diet.

Many people find that they can tolerate foods to which they are sensitive if they eat them no more than once every four or five days, and then not in excessive quantities. The plan below gives rotation suggestions, but you do not need to apply all of the suggestions. Stick to rotating the foods, or food groups, that are troubling you. So, for instance, if meat and vegetables do not give you any trouble, eat them freely whenever you wish. If grains, fish, some fruits and nuts are troublesome, rotate them as suggested in the plan, or make your own plan. In order to avoid wasting food, or being tempted to snack on foods you ate the previous day, cook only as much as you need for that day or freeze any leftovers (assuming they are suitable for freezing).

Ideally, you need to eat foods in their unadulterated form because composite foods will almost certainly catch you out with their ingredients, unless you make them at home. If you are using shop-bought composite foods, you need to be very aware of their ingredients, and try to buy high quality foods, otherwise they will inevitably contain ingredients which cross the lists. For instance, cake may have as its ingredients wheat (grains), milk (dairy), oil, eggs (fowl) and possibly fruit; or a burger may have beef (meat), soya flour (legume), onion (vegetables), egg (fowl). These might be fine to make for a particular day on your rotation plan, but usually make the exercise more complicated.

The advantage of the rotation diet is that it allows people with multiple food sensitivities to enjoy most foods to which they react on an occasional basis, and over time may tolerate more frequently. But don't be tempted to overdo it if you are feeling better, as this can put you straight back to square one.

	DAY 1	DAY 2
MEAT AND DAIRY	pork	venison
	bacon	
	sausages	
	goat's milk, cheese and yoghurt	
POULTRY AND GAME	turkey	duck
		goose and goose eggs
FISH	salmon	cod
	trout	haddock
	crab	coley
	lobster	
	prawns	
GRAINS	wheat	rice
	barley	sago

Following a rotation diet is not considered a good idea when undergoing enzyme potentiated desensitisation (see **Desensitisation**, page 180), and foods to which you react anaphylactically should not, of course, be eaten in any circumstances – even on a rotation basis.

Use the following as a guide only, and remember that, ideally, you should also avoid eating foods from the same families on consecutive days (see **Food Families**, page 164). All the food groups have been represented, to enable you to avoid falling into the pitfall of ending up on a nutritionally depleted diet.

DAY 3	DAY 4	DAY 5
lamb	rabbit	beef
mutton	hare	veal
ewe's milk, cheese and yoghurt		cow's milk, cheese and yoghurt
grouse	chicken and hen's eggs	pigeon
guineafowl	pheasant	
	partridge	
	quail	
snapper	mackerel	anchovy
octopus	tuna	clams
squid		mussels
		oysters
rye	millet	oats
quinoa	corn	buckwheat

	DAY 1	DAY 2
VEGETABLES	crucifer family: broccoli, cabbage, cauliflower, etc	squashes: cucumber, courgette, marrow, pumpkin, etc
	carrot family: celery, parsnip, fennel, etc	avocado
	peas	yam
FRUIT	blackcurrants	apple
	blueberry	melon
	cranberry	pear
	gooseberry	
NUTS AND SEEDS	hazelnuts	brazils
	sunflower seeds	pumpkin seeds
OILS	sunflower	groundnut (peanut)
DRINKS	juices made with fruit of the day	juices made with fruit of the day
	blackcurrant tea	apple and cinnamon tea
	fennel tea	redbush tea
TREATS	chocolate	honey
	wine	

DAY 3	DAY 4	DAY 5
composite: artichoke, lettuce, chicory, endive, etc mushrooms/Quorn lentils	nightshade family: potato, aubergine, peppers, tomatoes lily family: onion, leek, asparagus,etc soya	spinach family: beetroot, chard sweet potato beans
cherry peach plum prune	blackberry papaya raspberry strawberry	citrus grapes mango pineapple raisins
almonds	walnuts	cashews sesame seeds
olive	corn	sesame
juices made with fruit of the day rosehip tea black tea green tea	juices made with fruit of the day raspberry tea chamomile tea	juices made with fruit of the day lemon and hot water mint tea
carob beer	honey	coffee gin

Exclusion Diets

Usually, it is enough just to work out which food or foods may be contributing to your allergy or sensitivity problem, and then to exclude them. Relief from symptoms will underscore the correct diagnosis. As long as you are able to pick an alternative from within the same food group, you will not suffer any nutritional deficiencies as a result of giving up the food in question.

It is not, however, always possible to accurately pinpoint which foods might be the culprits (if indeed foods are involved at all), and in these circumstance the more rigorous approach of an exclusion diet is needed. Only embark on an exclusion diet if the low-allergy plan (see page 67) is not working for you.

An exclusion diet is purely and simply a diagnostic tool, the aim of the exercise being to find out which foods might be involved in your allergy reactions. An exclusion diet should never be followed for any length of time, as nutritional deficiencies can result. If you are under medical supervision for any reason you must check with your doctor to find out if following an exclusion diet for a limited period is acceptable. If it isn't, you must follow the more hit-and-miss approach of eliminating foods individually, and then reintroducing them to see if symptoms are either resolved or re-triggered. Children should not follow an exclusion diet in any circumstances without expert help from a paediatric dietician, nutritionist or doctor.

Before outlining the two exclusion diets, it is worth highlighting a few points:

● You may find that your symptoms improve after only a few

days, or you may have to be patient and wait two or three
weeks. If no improvement is felt after three weeks, you
may either be doing the exclusion diet incorrectly or foods
are not involved.

- It is not unusual for symptoms to get worse in the first few
  days of an exclusion diet, and you may even experience
  symptoms that you have not encountered before. You may
  find that headaches are bad for a couple of days (and in
  severe cases for up to five days) or you may get an
  unpleasant taste in your mouth, bad breath, a coated
  tongue, frequent urination, cloudy urine, altered bowel
  habits, fatigue and feel you need to rest.

- It may be wise to prepare for an exclusion diet two weeks
  in advance by taking a high strength vitamin and mineral
  supplement that gives 100 mg of B-vitamins, 15 mg of zinc,
  10 mg of iron, 300 mg each of calcium and magnesium, as
  well as a broad range of other vitamins and minerals, such as
  the antioxidants A, C, E and selenium. During the exclusion
  diet you must not take any supplements, as many contain
  colouring agents, or you may be sensitive to some of the
  ingredients. Nutritional supplements need to be tested for
  reactions in the same way as foods.

- For the reasons given above, it is best to avoid medication
  during an exclusion diet, but you must consult your doctor
  to ascertain if you are able to come off any prescribed
  drugs.

- You must not continue on an exclusion diet indefinitely as
  it is unhealthy to do so – an exclusion diet is for diagnosis
  only and not for treatment.

- You are likely to lose a lot of weight during the course of
  an exclusion diet, so if you are already underweight it is
  not advisable to go on such a regime.

- Allow sufficient time to see the exclusion diet through. A badly performed exclusion diet is useless. In the worst cases you may need to allow six weeks to test foods fully, and so planning to start a programme such as this just before Christmas or some other holiday is probably doomed to failure. Ideally, start the diet on a Friday so that if you have unpleasant symptoms, such as headaches, you are able to rest quietly at home over the weekend.

KEEPING A DIARY

It is a good idea to keep a diary during your exclusion diet, and during the phase when you reintroduce foods. Be methodical about this and it will pay dividends. Make columns to list meals and foods eaten. On a separate column make a note of how you feel overall that day, what your sleeping patterns are, if you experience any symptoms, if you get through the day without any symptoms or if you experience any new symptoms. Be careful to note the timing of any symptoms you experience in order that you can go back at a later date to see if this tallies with any foods eaten and if a pattern emerges. Use highlighter pens to mark out any events of particular interest.

THE LAMB AND PEARS DIET

This is a highly successful exclusion diet and is the simplest, though also the most boring and restrictive, to follow. You may eat only the following foods:

● Lamb – this includes grilled, roasted or casseroled (with pear slices) meat, liver, kidneys and sweetbreads. If you do not like lamb, turkey and turkey liver can be used as alternatives. Organic meat is preferable to non-organic meat (particularly in the case of turkey) but is not essential.

● Pears – without the skins, and make sure they are not mouldy or overripe. Freshly made pear juice, diluted with water, makes a refreshing drink.

● Bottled still mineral (not spring) water.

This exclusion diet must only be followed for five to seven days, after which you begin to reintroduce foods (see page 149).

THE MODIFIED EXCLUSION DIET

This exclusion diet is much easier to follow. The list below details which foods are to be eaten, and which are to be avoided. The diet should be followed until symptoms resolve (either partially or totally) for a maximum of three weeks. If your symptoms resolve in a shorter time – say within seven to ten days – you may start reintroducing foods after that time (though be cautious about symptoms which are intermittent as you may just be going through a 'clear' period. If you get migraines fortnightly, being migraine-free for one week does not necessarily indicate that the exclusion diet is working). The foods to eat and avoid are as follows:

	You can eat	You must avoid
MEAT AND POULTRY	lamb turkey game rabbit	chicken beef pork, bacon sausages preserved meats
FISH	white fish (unless you have eczema)	all other fish smoked fish shellfish

	You can eat	You must avoid
DAIRY PRODUCTS	none (rice milk may be used as a dairy substitute)	all (including yoghurt, butter, goat and ewe milk products, and soya milk)
CEREALS	rice, ground rice, rice flakes, rice flour, rice cakes, rice crispies buckwheat, millet, tapioca, sago	all others, including wheat, oats, barley, rye and corn

VEGETABLES	all vegetables and beans
	(pulses) other than
	those on the 'avoid'
	list
		potatoes, aubergines,
		   peppers
		onions, garlic
		sweetcorn
		soya
		broad beans
		green beans
		if you have bowel
		   problems also avoid
		   beans, lentils, cabbage
		   and Brussels sprouts

FRUIT	bananas, pears, mangoes, pomegranates, papayas	all other fruit, including tomatoes
FATS	cold pressed sunflower oil, safflower oil, olive oil, flax oil	corn oil, soya oil, mixed vegetable oil, nut oils, groundnut (peanut) oil, margarines, butter

	You can eat	You must avoid
DRINKS	filtered, bottled mineral, or distilled water	tea, coffee, fruit squashes, juices from fruits not allowed (particularly orange or grapefruit juice), alcohol, unfiltered tap water
	juices made from allowed fruits (half and half with hot water for a warm drink)	
	vegetable juices made from allowed vegetables	
MISCELLANEOUS	sea salt	chocolate, yeast, preservatives, food additives (see pages 172-5), herbs, spices, sugar, honey

REINTRODUCING FOODS

If you are on a restricted diet, such as the one above, it makes sense to reintroduce foods that are relatively safe first – mainly meat, vegetables, fruit, herbs and spices. It is best to keep the most suspicious foods until later on in the reintroduction plan.

The ideal order in which to reintroduce foods you have been avoiding is as follows, bearing in mind that you will have been eating some of these foods on the modified exclusion diet, but not on the lamb (or turkey) and pears diet:

● tap water
● beef, pork, 100 per cent pork or beef sausages

- chicken, eggs
- fish, oily and white
- rice, millet, corn, sweetcorn
- fruit other than citrus fruit
- tomatoes, potatoes, aubergine, peppers
- citrus fruit and juices
- nuts (other than peanuts)
- rye, barley, oats
- soya milk, tofu, legumes, peanuts
- milk, goat's milk products, sheep's milk products, white cheese, yellow cheese, blue cheese, butter
- yeast (6 brewer's yeast tablets or 2 teaspoons of baker's yeast)
- wheat (wholemeal spaghetti or soda bread to avoid yeast), couscous, spelt (yeast free), sprouted wheat
- alcohol, sugar, plain chocolate, tea, coffee

Introduce the less suspicious foods at a rate of two or three a day, but the more suspicious ones more slowly – one food a day, or even one food every two days. Within each group of foods treat each major type of food as a separate food. In other words, introduce milk, white cheese, yellow cheese, blue cheese, goat's milk and sheep's milk all separately. Do not at any time introduce foods that you know might lead to anaphylaxis.

Introduce foods in normal size portions. If you eat just a taste of the food you may find that symptoms are missed; excessive portions are equally unhelpful. A normal portion is a glass of milk, two slices of bread or 100 g of meat or beans.

When you reintroduce a food you may find that you get a reaction, such as hives or stomach pains, a short time after eating, a few hours afterwards or even, in the case of arthritis or muscle aches, up to three days later. If you get a reaction to a food, stop eating it to allow any symptoms to settle down before going on to reintroduce another food. If you are uncertain whether a food has caused a reaction, treat it as suspicious and avoid it anyway. You may want to experiment again with the suspect food at a later date to see if you can duplicate your reaction.

The object of the exercise is to return to as normal a diet as possible, as soon as you can after you have identified any foods to which you are sensitive. If you find that you are sensitive to a large number of foods, it is advisable to seek professional nutritional help in order to avoid ending up with too restricted a diet. For the most part, you should be able to find enjoyable alternatives to foods that you have to avoid or restrict. It may take a little getting used to, and you may need to be a bit more creative with your meal plans, but it is worth it if you no longer suffer from asthma, eczema, migraines or whatever is ailing you!

COMMON SOURCES OF FOOD INGREDIENTS AND THEIR ALTERNATIVES

If you need to avoid foods that are pretty much staples of your diet, it helps if you are well prepared with alternatives. Once you get used to eating some of the alternatives, it becomes quite easy. It is a question of creating new habits, and you'll be surprised how quickly you get used to reaching into the cupboard for rye crackers or oatcakes instead of wheat biscuits. You will also need to get used to buying different foods in your local supermarket or deli. Where once you might have automatically reached for the sandwiches, you need to create new buying habits. Learn to reach for the soups, salads, sushi, dips or other treats you enjoy and other choices with which you are comfortable.

A common complaint of many people is that they do not care for the alternatives because they are unused to the taste of them. Nobody would suggest that avoiding foods should mean eating those that you do not enjoy, but you need to abide by a few ground rules, otherwise it becomes too easy to give up at the first hurdle. First of all, give it a fair chance. Yes, soya milk and rice cakes taste different. But learn how to use them and what they go with, and soon you might find that you enjoy them. For instance, soya milk makes a particularly creamy porridge and is excellent in desserts, while rice cakes taste best spread with nut butters or piled high with seafood or dressed salad vegetables. Also make a point of tasting different brands of various foods, because they really do offer different options and tastes. You may also need to brush up on your cooking skills. It is fine for me to say that barley, quinoa and millet grains are all terrific substitutes for rice, but until you experiment with them you will just have to take my word for it! Finally, if you do decide to try something new, you will be surprised at how quickly your tastes change.

Avoiding dairy foods

Cow's milk and cheeses are detrimental for many people with allergies, particularly those with respiratory allergies. Milk contains casein, a protein that is difficult to digest, and which encourages excess mucus production. While dairy products are a good source of calcium, they are low in magnesium, a mineral needed for proper calcium absorption and for nerve control of the smooth muscle of the lungs, digestive tract and other regions of the body. Calcium-enriched alternatives to milk are widely available for those who are concerned about not getting enough of the mineral in their diet.

In addition to the obvious – i.e. milk, cheese, yoghurt – dairy products can crop up in cakes, breads, cereals, desserts, confectionery and restaurant prepared food (such as scrambled eggs, cream sauces, soufflés, soups, creamed potatoes).

Rice milk	A sweet tasting milk which is good on cereals and in milky drinks, but not much good in tea or coffee.
Soya milk	A very versatile alternative which is ideal for adding to cereals and porridge and is excellent when used in cooking. A high proportion of dairy-intolerant people are also sensitive to soya.
Soya yoghurt	The type with live bacteria is the best to use. Fruit flavoured soya yoghurts usually have a fair amount of sugar added.
Soya cheese	Best used for grilling on top of dishes.
Tofu	A tasteless soya bean curd block available in firm or soft textures that takes on the taste of the dish to which it is added. Used in stir-frys, marinated for kebabs or sandwiches, cubed into soups or fruit salads. Silken tofu is ideal to use instead of milk in 'milk' shakes.
Oat milk	Usually very well tolerated and ideal for cooking and on cereals. Oat yoghurt is also available.
Coconut milk	This creamy milk is best diluted by at least half. It makes a delicious substitute for cream in dessert dishes. Coconut and other nut creams are also available from better health food shops.
Almond milk	Available from health food shops and excellent in desserts as well as savoury dishes.
Goat's and sheep's milk	Goat's and sheep's milk, yoghurt and cheeses can often be tolerated by people with a cow's milk allergy. Exclude them

during an avoidance period for dairy products, but when you reintroduce them you may well find that they are well tolerated.

Alternatives to wheat

The grain that causes the most allergy problems is wheat. Wheat is found, principally, in bread, pasta, cereals, crackers, biscuits, savoury snacks, flours, pastries, breaded products, desserts, sausages and soups. If an ingredient listing mentions starch, it is often wheat-based.

Many people who need to avoid wheat find that they can eat other gluten-containing grains and products – oats, rye, barley, spelt, couscous and sprouted wheat – though it is best not to eat these during an initial two-week avoidance phase to test for sensitivities.

If you are in the habit of adding wheat bran to your food to keep yourself 'regular', you will need to substitute either oat bran or gluten-free alternatives such as rice bran, linseeds or psyllium husks. The last two rarely cause allergy problems.

Oats There are many oat and oat-based products available, including porridge oats, oatcakes, oat flapjacks and oat biscuits, but check the labels to make sure that they do not also contain wheat. Oats are particularly good used as a crunchy topping for sweet and savoury baked pies. Whole rolled oats can easily be made into a flour in your food processor.

Rye In the Middle Ages rye was widely used in England to make a firm textured bread, and in Eastern Europe they continue to make it today. It is difficult, but not impossible, to find 100 per cent rye bread in bakeries and supermarkets in the UK. It is often combined with wheat flour and, generally speaking, the lighter the colour and texture of the bread the more wheat flour it contains. Dark, flat 'German' rye bread and pumpernickel bread is readily available and has a slightly sour, but pleasant, taste. One hundred per cent rye crackers are also widely available, just check the label to make sure they don't contain wheat. Rye can cross-react with wheat antibodies and some wheat-intolerant people will find they need to avoid rye as well.

Barley This is a much underused grain, usually only put in winter stews. It can, however, be cooked and served in the same way as rice, and served as a side dish, added to salads or used as a base for a variety of dishes.

Spelt This is an old strain of wheat, which many people who need to avoid modern wheat find they can tolerate. It can be used in the same way as normal wheat flour. Occasionally you can find 100 per cent spelt flour bread in speciality shops. Must be avoided during the avoidance phase.

Tricale A cross between wheat and rye, which is sometimes tolerated. It is available as flakes and flour. Must be avoided during the avoidance phase.

Couscous This is also made from wheat, but again a different type which may be tolerated by those avoiding modern wheats. It cooks very quickly by steaming, making it a delicious fast food. It must be avoided during the avoidance phase.

Sprouted wheat Bread made from sprouted wheat grains, which has a delicious chewy texture, is available from health food shops. Make sure the product doesn't contain any ordinary wheat flour. Because the grain has been sprouted, it loses some of its allergenic potential for some people. Must be avoided during the avoidance phase.

Gluten-free grains

It is quite possible to find that all the gluten grains listed above cause sensitivity problems. The non-gluten grains, however, tend not to cause reactions (other than corn, which occasionally does). Here are the options to experiment with.

Rice A very familiar grain, available in many different strains, though brown rice is always a better source of fibre and nutrients. If you find cooking brown rice seems to take too long, try making a bigger batch than you need – it keeps well in the refrigerator for three days, or you can freeze portion sizes. Rice cakes, rice flour, rice pasta, rice puffs and Chinese rice crackers (a great snack) are all useful store cupboard stand-bys.

Corn This is the most common allergy-causing grain in the US, but it can be well-tolerated if exposure to it is limited. There are many corn products available, including maize meal (polenta flour), corn flour, cornflakes, sweetcorn, popcorn, corn pasta, tortillas and nachos, as well as recipes for corn bread and cakes based on maize. See **Avoiding Corn** below.

Quinoa An Andean 'grain', which is not a grain at all, but it cooks like one and and can be used as a substitute for rice or be mixed in with it. It makes a good base for filling salads when served cold, and can be used as an alternative to couscous.

Buckwheat Despite its name, this is not related to wheat at all.

Buckwheat flour, pasta and noodles are all readily available, though the latter, which are the basis for many Japanese noodle dishes, are best bought from health food shops, and you need to check the labels to ensure they are wheat-free. The flour can be made into Russian blinis – flat, bready pancakes that are useful alternatives to bread. They can be interleaved with baking parchment, frozen and then taken out and popped into a toaster as needed.

Millet Often thought of as bird food, millet is in fact very nutritious. The whole grain can be cooked like rice. It is also available as flakes, which can be made into porridge or muesli.

Potato A useful starchy base to a meal if you are avoiding grains. Baked potatoes are the most nutritious, and if you are roasting or steaming leave the skins on in order to benefit from their nutrients and fibre. Potato flour can be used to thicken sauces or, using another, non-gluten flour alongside it, to make potato cakes.

Sweet potato Another useful root vegetable, which has even more fibre in it than potato. It can be cooked in all the various ways that potato can. Yams can also be used in the same way.

Legumes Beans of all description make a filling base to many meals, including soups and salads.

Chestnuts Chestnut flour can be used as a thickening agent or added to other flours to change the texture or taste.

Sago Made from the pith of palm and used for puddings.

Tapioca This comes from the cassava plant, and is available as hard round grains or ground into a flour. It is used as a thickening agent or for puddings.

Gram Gram flour, made from chick peas, is readily available from Indian (or similar) shops and is used in many Indian recipes. Lentil flour (used to make popadums) is also available.

Avoiding corn

Occasionally, corn presents a problem and, because it is found in so many foods, it can be a little complicated to avoid. Corn flour, corn syrup and corn oil are all used extensively in food processing. Even glucose and dextrose (sugars) are usually made from corn.

Apart from the obvious – cornflakes, popcorn, polenta, tortillas – foods that often contain corn include: cereals which list corn syrup as an ingredient, cakes, biscuits, desserts, baking powders, custard powder, sauces, sweets made from corn syrup, margarines and vegetable oils, carbonated drinks (which use corn syrup as a sweetener), jams, sauces, even toothpastes and sticky labels.

Avoiding soya

Soya is also used extensively in the food processing industry, and it is a fairly common allergenic food. The obvious soya-containing foods are soya milk, soya yoghurt, soy sauce and tamari. Soya is also used in soya flour and TVP (textured vegetable protein), which find their way into a vast number of processed foods. These include most commercially made breads, pastries and cakes. In addition, many processed meats, pastas, salad dressings, sauces, sweets and margarines contain soya oil. Quorn is not soya-based.

Avoiding yeast

There are two main types of yeast listed on food labels, baker's yeast and brewer's yeast. Yeasts and moulds are found in all of the following:

- most breads, including flat breads such as pitta bread and pizza bases
- bread sauce, breaded foods such as fish fingers, fish cakes, breaded chicken, vegeburgers, pizza
- commercially made pies and puddings containing bread
- most cheeses, buttermilk, sour cream, synthetic cream (enjoy yoghurt and cottage cheese)
- yeast extracts (such as Marmite), stock cubes, beef extract
- dried fruit, overripe or mouldy fruit, grapes, fruit juices other than freshly squeezed
- vinegar (use lemon instead), sauerkraut, pickles, ketchups, salad creams
- malted drinks
- mushrooms, Quorn
- foods left out in warm or moist conditions for any length of time (refrigerate all foods or eat shortly after opening packages to avoid this problem)
- brewer's yeast supplements, many B-vitamin supplements and many chromium supplements.

Brewer's yeast is found in all fermented alcoholic drinks such as beer, wine and whisky. Those which are filtered, however, such as vodka and gin, may be tolerated.

Breads and crackers that are usually yeast-free (though check the labels) include: chappatis, Matzos, traditionally baked scones, soda bread, oatcakes, popadums and Ryvita. You can use baking powder instead of yeast to make soda bread and also make pancakes, dumplings and crumbles.

Sugar in the diet can promote the growth of yeasts within the gut, and ideally sugars and refined carbohydrates should be avoided. For suggestions on sugar alternatives see below, and instead of eating refined carbohydrates concentrate on eating whole grains, such as whole porridge oats, rye-based products, brown wholegrain rice and quinoa.

Alternatives to sugar

Sugar does not cause allergy reactions, but it is so successful at undermining blood sugar control, adrenal health and digestive and immune health that it is closely implicated in the whole allergy problem. Sugar also promotes yeast infections. There are many alternative names to look out for on ingredients lists: sucrose, glucose, dextrose, lactose, fructose, corn syrup, golden syrup and the term malted. Foods which contain high amounts of sugar include confectionery, jams, honey, desserts, flavoured yoghurts, ice cream, maple syrup, chocolate, figs, dates, cakes, biscuits, cereals, squashes, some juices, 'energy' drinks, and many tinned and packaged foods.

Because artificial sweeteners can trigger allergy-type reactions in some people, it is best to satisfy your craving for sweetness by being more creative with sweet tasting fruits. Use chopped dried fruit (preferably unsulphured) on cereals and when baking, experiment with puréed fruits (fresh and dried) as sauces and drink diluted fresh fruit juices. If you are not sensitive to it, a little 70 per cent cocoa solids chocolate grated on top of a dish, or a couple of cubes as a dessert, goes a long way towards satisfying the urge for something sweet. A little honey can also make life sweeter and manuka honey from New Zealand is particularly known for its antibiotic, immune stimulating properties.

Fructose, even though it is a (fruit) sugar, does not have such a detrimental impact on blood sugar levels as ordinary sugar, and is thus a good alternative for many people when used in moderation, particularly as it works well in hot drinks. It is easy to find in health food shops. Another option is to use is FOS (fructo-oligo-saccharides), a sweet tasting powder which encourages healthy bowel bacteria and is available from various supplement companies and health shops. FOS is good on cereals, OK in hot drinks, but not ideal for cooking. As it is a fibre it can take some getting used to and may cause bloating initially. Start off at a low level of a teaspoon or two daily and build up to a couple of tablespoons daily if you wish – one of those rare instances where you can have your sweetness since it is good for you.

Avoiding eggs

Eggs are a common ingredient in manufactured foods, making them hard to avoid. In some people the tiniest amount can lead to a serious reaction, others have an intolerance which requires a larger amount to cause a reaction, for example eating one egg a day. If you suspect an egg intolerance or allergy these are things to look out for:

- Sometimes well-cooked egg is tolerated whereas soft cooked egg is not. This is because the cooking changes the protein structure.
- Other types of eggs may also cause a reaction, including

duck and quail's eggs. On the other hand, some people who are sensitive to hen's eggs find that they can eat other types.

- Some people are sensitive to both hen's eggs and to chicken meat (this is rare and relates mostly to hens and not to male chickens).

- Severely egg allergic people need to avoid ingredients listed as: eggs, egg white, lecithin (E322), meringue, albumin, canalbumin, ovalbumin, ovamucin and ovaglobulin.

- Foods which commonly contain eggs include: foods in breadcrumbs or batter, baby foods and cereals, biscuits, breads, cakes, chocolate, creams, dessert toppings, ice cream and sorbets, lemon curd, marshmallows, macaroons, meringue, mayonnaise, noodles, pasta, pastries, processed meat, puddings, ready-prepared desserts, salad dressings, sauces, soups, stock cubes, sweets and wines that have been clarified using egg white.

- Some live-virus vaccines, such as measles and influenza, are grown in chick embryos or egg culture and can provoke a reaction in sensitive people.

If you need to avoid eggs, you can get 'egg-replacer' from many health food shops, though check the label as some products are in fact pasteurised dried egg white or whole egg (this applies also to leading brands available from supermarkets). It does not produce particularly successful omelettes or meringues, but does make good pancakes.

Eggs are used for a variety of reasons in cooking and finding substitutes for them is easier if you understand what you are aiming to achieve.

If you use eggs for	instead use
thickening	2 tablespoons of cornflour or arrowroot in place of each egg used.
glazing	Milk or soya milk, brushed on top of pasties or bread before baking
binding	For savoury dishes such as burgers, croquettes and rissoles, use tomato purée, mashed potato, moistened breadcrumbs or moistened rolled oats; other possibilities include 1 tablespoon tahini, or 1 tablespoon soya flour per egg used, mixed to a paste with water.
	For sweet dishes such as biscuits and muffins use half a mashed banana, 25 g mashed tofu, 25 g apple sauce or 12 g prune purée for each egg used.
their raising properties	1 teaspoon bicarbonate of soda with ½ teaspoon cream of tartar, or use 1 teaspoon baking powder. Alternatively, dissolve 1 tablespoon agar-agar in 1 tablespoon of water and whisk thoroughly.

Egg-free 'mayonnaise' can also be made using soya milk, nut milk or tofu.

Alternatives to potato

Potatoes are both filling and versatile, and many people cannot imagine a meal without them. Once you try, however, it is relatively easy to centre a meal on other starches, such as rice, quinoa, buckwheat or millet. Alternatively, you can use baked sweet potatoes, yams, and roasted or mashed root vegetables (which are also excellent used as toppings for savoury pies such as fish or shepherd's pie). Potato flour is often used as a thickener and starch in processed foods, so you need to check ingredients lists.

FOOD FAMILIES

Foods belong to families, some of whose members can be surprising. It is odd to think, for instance, that the date belongs to the same family as the coconut, the palm family, or that bamboo and wheat are related, but they are both grasses.

There can be a certain amount of cross-reaction between members of the same food family. This does not necessarily mean, however, that if you have an allergy to a particular food you will automatically also be allergic to all the other members of that family. It is quite possible to have a strong allergy to, say, tomatoes and yet be able to eat potatoes quite happily. You may find that eggs cause a problem yet chicken is fine, and that dairy produce induces symptoms whereas beef is OK. Nevertheless, when working out which foods may be causing your adverse reactions, it is as well to be suspicious of foods in the same family until you can eliminate them as culprits.

Plant families

applo	apple, pear, quince
avocado	avocado, cinnamon
banana	arrowroot, banana, plantain
beechnut	beechnut, chestnut
pepper	black pepper, white pepper
blueberry	blueberry, cranberry
buckwheat	buckwheat, rhubarb
carrot	anise, carrot, caraway, celery, coriander, cumin, dill, fennel, parsnip, parsley
cashew	cashew, mango, pistachio
citrus	citron, clementine, grapefruit, kumquat, lemon, lime, orange, tangerine, ugli
coffee	coffee
cola	chocolate, cola
composite	chamomile, chicory, dandelion, endive, globe artichoke, goldenrod, Jerusalem artichoke, lettuce, safflower, salsify, sunflower, tarragon
crucifer	broccoli, Brussels sprouts, cabbage, cauliflower, Chinese leaves, collards, cress, horseradish, kale, kohlrabi, mustard, rape, turnip, swede (rutabaga)
elderberry	elderberry
ginger	ginger, turmeric
ginseng	American and Korean (not Siberian)
grape	currants, grapes, raisins, sultanas
grass	bamboo, barley, corn, millet, oats, rice, rye, sugar cane, wheat
guava	allspice, clove, guava
lily	asparagus, chives, garlic, leek, shallot, onion
lychee nut	lychee
macadamia	macadamia nut

maple	maple syrup
mint	basil, lavender oil, majoram, peppermint, rosemary, sage, spearmint, thyme
mulberry	breadfruit, fig, mulberry
mushroom	mushrooms (fungi, Quorn)
nightshade	aubergine, capsicum, tobacco, tomato, peppers (sweet and hot), potato
nutmeg	mace, nutmeg
okra	okra (bindi)
palm	coconut, date, sago
papaya	papaya
persimmon	persimmon
pineapple	pineapple
plum	almond, apricot, cherry, greengage, peach, plum, prune
pulses (legumes)	beans, lentils, liquorice, pea, peanut, soya (tofu)
quinoa	quinoa
sarsaparilla	sarsaparilla
saxifrage	blackcurrant, gooseberry, redcurrant
spinach	beetroot, chard, spinach, sugar beet
squash	cucumber, courgette (zucchini), marrow, melon, pumpkin, squash, watermelon
strawberry	blackberry, strawberry, raspberry
sweet potato	sweet potato
tapioca	tapioca
tea	black tea, green tea
vanilla	vanilla
walnut	hickory, pecan, walnut
water chestnut	water chestnut

Animal families

crustacea	crab, crayfish, lobster, prawn, shrimp
fish (main families)	anchovy
	bass, grouper, mullet
	carp
	catfish
	cod, coley, haddock, hake, whiting
	conger eel
	eel
	sturgeon
	dab, flounder, halibut, plaice, sole, turbot
	herring, pilchard, sprat, shad
	bonito, mackerel, tuna
	pike
	snapper
	salmon, trout
molluscs	clam, mussel, oyster, scallop
	abalone, conch, snail
	octopus, squid
cattle	beef, buffalo, goat, lamb, mutton, milk and dairy products from beef, buffalo, goat or sheep
deer	deer, elk, venison
duck	duck, goose and their eggs
grouse	grouse, guineafowl, turkey and their eggs
pheasant	chicken, pheasant, partridge, peafowl, quail and their eggs
pig	bacon, ham, gammon, pork
pigeon	pigeon and pigeon's eggs
rabbit	hare, rabbit

FOOD ADDITIVES

There are many excellent books about additives and the adverse reactions they can cause in some people (see **Resources**, page 195). Since there isn't space here to detail all the ones that can cause problems, I have only listed below those that are generally considered to be OK. It is a much shorter list!

By and large, government agencies and food manufacturers adopt the line that all additives that have been approved for use are safe. However, the problem with such a broad approach as this is that individual cases of sensitivity are missed. There is sufficient evidence to suggest that sensitive people can suffer a worsening of symptoms such as asthma, eczema, hyperactivity, insomnia and urticaria when exposed to some food additives.

Adverse reactions to food additives, including asthma, eczema, urticaria and childhood hyperactivity, have been described in a number of research papers. Reactions to the dye tartrazine (E102) and its related compounds (most of the E compounds between E103–155), which are used in desserts, jellies and squashes, to benzoates (E210–219), the antioxidants BHA and BHT (E320–321), and to the sulphite preservatives (E220–228), which are used in wine production and squashes, are often reported. Sulphite compounds frequently cause asthma problems. People who are sensitive to aspirin, which is common in asthma, may also be sensitive to the benzoates or tartrazine.

Some additives that are currently allowed in the UK are banned in Finland, Norway, Australia, the USA and Japan. Just as worryingly, many of the colourings which are banned in other countries, such as E104 (quinoline yellow), E110 (sunset yellow) and E124 (ponceau 4R or red No 4), and which were voluntarily removed from products aimed at children a few years ago after concerns about hyperactivity and cancer were raised, have now crept back.

One way to avoid preservatives is to buy freshly-made food and freeze it, or to buy preservative-free frozen foods, since frozen food should not need preservatives (though check the labels).

Remember to be cautious about medicines and supplements in highly coloured capsules, or medicinal syrups. Good quality vitamin and mineral supplements should use natural food colourings, such as anthocyanidins, but many use additives that may trigger allergic symptoms. Discuss with your doctor any prescribed drugs which are in coloured capsules, and about which you are concerned. Also be wary about the term 'natural flavourings' on packages, as this can include salicylates (see pages 176-7) or MSG (monosodium glutamate or E621).

Generally, the real baddies, in terms of adverse reactions, are the colours E102–180, especially the azo dyes, which include tartrazine, sunset yellow and amaranth, though, as you will see from the list below, there are some that are OK as they are based on natural colourings.

The following list has been condensed from a mini-guide available from Foresight, which in turn was abridged from *E for Additives* by Maurice Hanssen. If an additive is not on the list, you should treat it with suspicion.

Colourings

E100	curcumin
E101	riboflavin
E140	chlorophyll
E160	carotene
E161	lutein and xanthins
E162	beetroot
E163	anthocyanins
E170	calcium carbonate (chalk)
E172	iron oxides

Preservatives

E234	nisin
E260	acetic acid
E262	sodium diacetate
E263	calcium acetate
E290	carbon dioxide (promotes effects of alcohol)
E297	fumaric acid

Antioxidants

E300–304	ascorbates (vitamin C)
E306–309	tocopherols (vitamin E)

Emulsifiers, stabilisers and others

E322	lecithins (unless soya or egg allergy)
E330–331	citrates
E335–337	tartrates
E350–352	malates
E353	metatartaric acid
E355	adipic acid
E363	succinic acid
E375	nicotinic acid (vitamin B3)
E400-405	alginates
E406	agar-agar
E440	pectin
E501	potassium carbonate
E503	ammonium carbonate
E504	magnesium carbonate
E516	calcium sulphate
E528	magnesium hydroxide
E551–552	silicas
E559	kaolin
E576	sodium gluconate
E577	potassium gluconate

E578	calcium gluconate
E901	beeswax
E903	carnauba wax
E907	microcrystalline wax

HISTAMINE-CONTAINING FOODS

In addition to being made in the body, histamine is generated by bacteria found in foods. Some people, including some asthmatics, are highly sensitive to histamine in foods and their livers may not be successful at neutralising it. High histamine foods can result in symptoms similar to allergy reactions, including asthma attacks. In some people, high histamine foods may result in reddening of the face (for instance after a glass or two of red wine) or rashes. The following foods are high in histamine:

- red wine (about 1000 mcg per litre)
- champagne (about 650 mcg per litre)
- dessert wine (about 300 mcg per litre)
- white, rosé and sparkling wines (35–50 mcg per litre)
- some beers, including non-alcoholic ones (20–30 mcg per litre)
- very ripe cheeses, such as Emmenthal and Gouda
- continental sausages (the kind that are found in Italy and Spain and which are cured for years before eating)
- fish such as mackerel or tuna, if not cooked or canned when very fresh
- pickled cabbage and other pickled foods

In addition to histamine-containing foods, some foods have a histamine releasing action. These include egg whites, shellfish, strawberries, tomatoes and chocolate.

LOW SALICYLATE DIET

Salicylates are substances found in many foods which are related to aspirin and which can trigger allergy reactions. Aspirin-induced asthma has been reported in up to 20 per cent of asthmatics, some of whom are sensitive to even small amounts (such as 30 mg), whereas in others quite a large dose (such as 300 mg) is needed to trigger an attack. Theoretically, if someone is sensitive to aspirin, then salicylates from foods may also pose a problem. Other conditions which often respond well to reducing salicylates in the diet include urticaria (nettle rash, hives), both acute and chronic, hyperactivity in children and, occasionally, allergic colitis.

Follow a two-week plan avoiding foods containing salicylates. Enjoy foods in the low-salicylate list freely. At the same time, avoid foods with artificial colours and flavourings and also medicines which contain aspirin (the chemical name for which is acetylsalicylic acid). Cross-reaction sensitivity with other analgesic (painkilling) drugs, such as ibuprofen, is fairly common.

Because a low-salicylate diet involves avoiding a number of foods which would normally be considered extremely healthy, such as broccoli and citrus fruit, this is not an approach to take unless absolutely necessary, and while some people respond very positively to this diet, not everyone does.

Low-salicylate food you can eat freely

fruits:	apples (not sharp tasting), banana, mango, passion fruit, papaya, pears (peeled), pomegranates
vegetables:	chick peas, dried beans (but not broad beans), bean sprouts, beetroot, Brussels sprouts, cabbage, carrots, leeks, lentils, lettuce, peas,

	potatoes (peeled), shallots, spinach, swede, sweetcorn, turnip
grains:	all cereals (apart from cornflour)
meats:	meats, fish, shellfish, eggs and dairy produce
nuts and seeds:	cashews, hazelnuts, pecans, poppy seeds, sunflower seeds
seasonings:	coriander leaves, garlic, fresh parsley, saffron, soy sauce, Tabasco, tamari, Tandoori powder, malt vinegar
miscellaneous:	herbal teas (unless on the avoid list of seasonings), decaffeinated tea
alcohol:	vodka

Salicylate containing foods to avoid

fruits:	raisins, prunes, apples (sharp, i.e. Granny Smiths), all berries (i.e. strawberries, blackberries, boysenberries, etc), citrus fruit, cherries, dried fruit, figs, guava, grapes (and currants, sultanas and raisins), kiwi, passion fruit, pineapple, apricots, dates, lychees, peaches, plums, prunes, plus jams and jellies made from these fruits
vegetables:	broccoli, chicory, endive, green beans, broad beans, mushrooms, peppers, radish, watercress, asparagus, avocado, cucumber (and gherkins and pickles), cauliflower, onion, tinned tomatoes, olives
meats:	sausages, frankfurters, salami, bologna and other cured meats
nuts and seeds:	almonds, pistachios, macadamia nuts, pine nuts, Brazil nuts, walnuts, coconut, peanuts, sesame seeds, water chestnuts

seasonings: Worcestershire sauce, aniseed, cayenne, celery
                   powder, cinnamon, curry powder, dill,
                   Chinese five spice, garam masala, mace,
                   mixed dried herbs, mustard, oregano,
                   paprika, rosemary, sage, tarragon, turmeric,
                   thyme, allspice, bayleaf, chilli, cloves,
                   ginger, mint, nutmeg, black pepper, pickles,
                   liquorice, peppermint, white pepper, plus
                   mouthwashes, etc, which use mint

miscellaneous: honey, chewing gum, tea, cornflour, coffee,
                   rose-hip, cornflour, diet drinks, cider
                   vinegar, soft drinks, yeasts, some ice
                   creams, some margarines, some cake mixes,
                   some speciality breads, some confectionery

alcohol: beer, cider, sherry, wine (red and white),
                   brandy, gin, rum, port, Tia Maria,
                   Benedictine, Drambuie

Salicylates, which may also be listed as salicylic acid, acetyl salicylic acid or ammonium salicylate, often turn up in other products which may cause reactions when you come into contact
with them, including:

●   suntan lotions
●   perfumes
●   cosmetics
●   soaps (wintergreen fragrance)
●   anti-mildew treatments
●   lubricating oils
●   plants such as tulips, violets, marigolds and camelias

URTICARIA PSEUDOALLERGEN FREE DIET

This diet is taken from one used in a trial* in which excellent results were achieved for people with chronic urticaria. It is pretty much based on the low-salicylate diet (see above) and strictly forbids all foods containing preservatives, dyes or commercial antioxidants, thus all industrially-processed foods should be regarded with suspicion. In practice, this means making all meals from scratch. Even prepared vegetables and salads may use preservatives, making them unsuitable. You also need to buy bread from a baker who you know does not use preservatives. Foods which may be sources of concealed pseudoallergens have been eliminated, for example colourants in eggs or in farmed salmon (which are fed canthaxanthin to imitate the colour of wild salmon).

For the first three days only freshly cooked, unsulphited potatoes, polished (white) rice, water and salt are allowed. For the next two weeks anything from the 'allowed' list can be eaten.

	Allowed	*Forbidden*
Basic Food	preservative-free bread, potatoes, rice, unprocessed cereals, flour	all others (e.g. noodles, potato chips)
Fat	butter, cold pressed plant oils	all others (e.g. margarine)

*The information in the chart above is taken from Zuberbier T. et al, Department of Dermatology, Humboldt Universität zu Berlin, Germany. *Pseudoallergen-free diet in the treatment of chronic urticaria*; Acta Derm Venereol (Stockh) 1995:75:484–7.

	Allowed	Forbidden
Milk Products	fresh milk, cream, white cheese, young Gouda	all others
Meat, Fish, Eggs	fresh meat	all others, including seafood
Vegetables	all, except those listed as forbidden	artichoke, peas, mushrooms, rhubarb, tomatoes, olives, sweet peppers
Fruits	none	all
Herbs, spices	salt, chives	all others
Sweets	none, except sugar and honey	all, including chewing gum
Beverages	milk, water, coffee, black tea	all others

In the trial, patients continued with the basic diet after the initial two weeks, but their diet was individually modified to include a wider range of foods which did not provoke reactions for them. After following the programme for two weeks you can begin to introduce foods one by one to see if they have any effect on your urticaria. It is best to wait 48 hours after introducing foods to establish whether or not you have a reaction (see page

149 for a suggested order in which to reintroduce foods). If you do not have a reaction continue to eat the food. It is possible that sensitivity to foods occur as a result of 'total load' and that urticaria, or other conditions, manifest when a threshold of eating certain groups or types of foods is reached. Being aware of this can help in the detective work if, and when, you get any reactions.

Allergy Tests

There are a number of allergy tests available, both through doctors and hospitals, as well as through private allergy laboratories and natural health practitioners. No test is perfect, some have merits, and some do not.

The most useful test is to avoid a food or foods and to then reintroduce them, to understand which symptoms respond and which return when a particular food is eaten again. However, there are times when laboratory tests have their uses.

Skin test

Also called an Intradermal or scratch test. A sublingual (under the tongue) test is also sometimes used. These are tests used by medical allergists. The prick and scratch test was developed in 1911 and has not changed significantly since then. It involves pricking or scratching the skin and applying the suspect substance, or injecting the substance under the skin. This test is used for inhaled and contact allergens and foods. If a red weal appears, the food is deemed to cause an allergic reaction. This test is subject to false readings, both false positive and false negative. In the case of foods this is not surprising, as it is not a normal route for allowing food into the body. Skin prick tests do not identify food intolerances. In the case of sublingual testing, a small amount of the suspect substance, usually a chemical, is placed under the tongue and the patient is then observed to see if they exhibit symptoms. After a reaction to one of these tests is observed, neutralisation may, in the case of inhaled allergens, be an option, though this is rarely successful with food allergens.

RAST

RAST (radioallergosorbent test) is a blood test that involves measuring the antibody response (IgE or IgG) to suspected food allergens with radioactive labels (for this reason there are environmental concerns about its use). It is quite effective, but not foolproof, and does not identify food intolerances. It is, however, a reasonably reliable way of discovering true allergies, and therefore the test has been adapted for use for food sensitivities. While this has improved the capacity to pick up non-allergic reactions, they are also susceptible to false positives.

ELISA

ELISA (enzyme-linked immuno-sorbent assay) is a blood test that measures the IgG antibody to around 100 foods. This test can have its uses and is becoming more accurate, but it may not be possible to replicate and the long list of foods reported with some of the ELISA test results can often lead to an unnecessarily restricted diet. My estimate is that ELISA can help about 70 per cent of the time.

Cytotoxic test

Cytotoxic testing looks at a sample of blood serum under a microscope to see if it reacts to up to 150 substances. The reliability of the result depends upon the laboratory being used, and on the abilities of the technician.

Cellular allergy test

This measures leukotriene responses to any foods. It is useful for true allergens as well as intolerances and, although it can give mixed results, it is probably more reliable than the ELISA test.

SIgA

This is another component of the immune response located in

the digestive tract. Increased levels of SIgA are produced when foods which irritate it are consumed. Testing for raised levels of SIgA can be a useful way of telling whether or not there is inflammation of the digestive tract lining, however it is non-specific about which foods might be causing the trouble. There is also a gliadin-SIgA which can identify if there is a problem with the gluten grains.

Kinesiology

This is a system of uncovering imbalances by testing the response of muscles to certain influences. Kinesiology uses a mixture of chiropractic muscle information and Chinese energy, or meridian, flows. The therapy is used for a number of health issues, including structural/muscular problems and emotional problems. As far as food testing is concerned, the theory is that certain foods, to which the individual is sensitive or intolerant, will interfere with the energy flows in the body and, at one level or another, interfere with muscle function. Nobody knows how this system really works, but work it does in many cases. This therapy is very dependent on the practitioner being experienced. In the hands of someone who knows what they are doing, it can be remarkably accurate, but if the practitioner is a novice it can be next to useless. Nevertheless, the 'biofeedback' from accurate testing can be very motivating.

Other tests

There are other testing methods available, but they are not particularly accurate and the results are difficult to replicate. These include pulse tests, hair and nail analysis, vega testing and dowsing.

Desensitisation

Desensitisation uses the same principles as mithridation, a process named after King Mithridates, a Persian ruler who protected himself against poisoning by his enemies. He took, over time, larger and larger doses of poison on a daily basis, until he could tolerate amounts that would normally kill someone. By slowly increasing exposure to the known allergen the body is tricked into accepting the substance and becomes desensitised.

Until the mid-1980s desensitisation injections for allergies, involving increasing exposure to the allergen, were commonly available in the UK but, after several fatalities from anaphylactic shock, were discontinued. The treatment is still available in other countries, but you should be aware of the potential dangers and exercise great caution before deciding to go ahead with it. In no circumstances should children be treated by this method.

An alternative option, which is also only available at specialised units with resuscitation equipment, is Enzyme Potentiated Desensitisation. This involves a course of 12 weekly injections of low doses of the allergen, say grass pollen extract for hay fever sufferers, or animal dander for asthmatics, along with other substances to increase the body's tolerance. This is followed by monthly injections for three years. The treatment becomes more effective each time and no fatalities have as yet been linked to it. Desensitisation treatments have not, however, proved successful in treating food allergies. Very few National Health Service doctors offer this facility and you would probably need to consult a private doctor specialising in allergies if you wished to try it.

There are also homeopathic desensitisation programmes available. Homeopathy involves 'potentising' a remedy to the point where there is only a chemical 'memory' of the original material used. Because of this it is generally very safe to use. Despite there being undetectable traces of the original compounds, homeopathy has proved itself time and time again, even with animals where a placebo effect cannot be claimed. Normally in homeopathy like heals like. This means that compounds are used which would elicit similar symptoms to those that need to be eradicated. In desensitisation there is a departure from this, and 'isopathy' is used where same heals same. In this instance, the substance that the person needs to be desensitised to is the substance which is potentised. Any substance can be potentised, including pollens, mixed moulds, wheat, milk, and even tap water, which is sometimes involved in health problems. Desensitisation is always best carried out by a medically qualified homeopath, and caution may be advised in some cases of asthma.

Glossary

allergen a substance such as pollen, cat hair or peanuts, which triggers an allergy

allergy an adverse response to a substance (see allergen) which triggers an allergic immune response

antibody a protein made in the body to disable and eliminate a 'foreign' body, such as a bacteria, virus or allergen

antigen a substance that triggers an immune response; an allergen is also an antigen but one that triggers an allergic reaction

antioxidants substances found in fruit and vegetables which neutralise damaging oxidation damage to body tissues. An allergic reaction results in oxidation damage

basophils cells which produce irritating histamine

DHA a fatty acid found in fish which may be helpful against the inflammation typical of allergic reactions

EPA a fatty acid found in fish which may be helpful against the inflammation typical of allergic reactions

GLA a fatty acid found in evening primrose and other oils which may be helpful against the inflammation typical of some allergic reactions

histamine an irritating chemical produced in the body which leads to redness and inflammation of tissues

IgE an immune compound involved in 'classic' allergies such as asthma, hay fever and peanut allergies

IgG an immune compound also involved in some types of adverse reactions to foods

intolerance a term used to describe adverse reaction to foods, which is sometimes associated with enzyme deficiency, as in lactose (milk sugar) intolerance, but which is also sometimes used when non-specific adverse reactions are noted

leukotrienes compounds made in the body from dietary fats, many of which cause a highly inflammatory reaction

mast cells cells which line the skin and mucus membranes and produce the irritating chemical, histamine

prostaglandins compounds made in the body from dietary fats, some of which increase inflammation, and some of which reduce inflammation

sensitivity (when applied to foods) an adverse reaction to foods which does not have a specific immune response explanation

steroids hormones produced by the adrenal glands which have an anti-inflammatory effect

Resources

To find out more about Suzannah Olivier's activities visit her website at:

www.healthandnutrition.co.uk

email: eattobefit@ aol.com

ALLERGY ASSOCIATIONS

BRITISH ALLERGY FOUNDATION
Helpline: 0891 516 500

ACTION AGAINST ALLERGY
Tel: 020 8303 8525

ANAPHYLAXIS CAMPAIGN
Tel: 01252 542 029
Website: www.anaphylaxis.org.uk

NATIONAL ASTHMA CAMPAIGN
Tel: 0845 701 0203

ECZEMA SOCIETY
Tel: 020 7388 344
Website: www.eczema.org

THE PSORIASIS ASSOCIATION
Tel: 01604 711 129

THE MIGRAINE TRUST
Tel: 020 7831 4818

NATIONAL SOCIETY FOR RESEARCH INTO ALLERGY
Tel: 01455 851 546

HERBAL AND NUTRIENT SUPPLEMENT SUPPLIES

BIOCARE
Birmingham Tel: 0121 433 3727
Stocked by good independent health food shops.
- Nutrients: large range of vitamins, minerals and antioxidant formulas.
- Essential fats: capsules – essential fatty acids, linseed oil, EPA, GLA, lipoplex; powder – range of essential fats, including salmon oil, pumpkin seed oil. Also caspules and Dricelle (powder) forms of MEGA GLA, EPO, linseed oil, omega 3.

BLACKMORES
Available from good quality health food shops.
- Nutrients: a full range of good quality herbs and nutrients.
- Essential fats: fish oil 1000.

EAST WEST HERB SHOP
Tel: 020 7379 1312
For Oriental herbs and mushroom supplements including the anti-histamine reishi.

ENZYMATIC THERAPY UK
Tel: 020 8449 1113
- Simcort cream for psoriasis.
- Laxseed oil in a blend with borage and pumpkin seed oils.

GNC (GENERAL NUTRITION COMPANY)

Tel: 01483 410 611

A wide range of nutritional products available by mail order and from their shops.

HEALTH PLUS

East Sussex Tel: 01323 492096

- Nutrients: range of nutrients. Also supply convenient daily dose packs, each containing a combination of supplements that are designed for specific health conditions. There are 28 daily packs in each box.
- Essential fats: EPO, starflower and fish oil, EPA, starflower oil, high strength starflower.

HIGHER NATURE

East Sussex Tel: 01435 882880

Direct mail-ordering service available.

- Nutrients: range of vitamins, minerals and antioxidant formulas.
- Essential fats: bottles of flaxseed oil (also chilli flavoured) and flavoured essential balance oil which are excellent alternatives to other salad oils. Ground linseeds, omega 3 fish oil capsules and starflower capsules.

LAMBERTS

Available from good independent health food retailers.

- Nutrients: range of vitamins, minerals and antioxidants formulas.
- Essential fats: capsules of Flaxseed oil, GLA, EPO, EPA.

NUTRI LTD

High Peak Tel: 0800 212742

- Nutrients: range of vitamins, minerals and antioxidants.

● Essential fats: Eskimo 3 capsules, Eskimo 3 liquid.

THE NUTRI CENTRE
London W1 Tel: 020 7436 5122

Stock an extensive range of nutrition products, including
NADH, health foods and books from various suppliers and
manufacturers. They also have their own range, NutriWest.
You can either visit their shop or obtain their stock by mail
order.

SAVANT DISTRIBUTION
Leeds Tel: 0113 2301993

● Fats and oils: almond oil, canola (rapeseed) oil, flaxseed
oil, pumpkin seed oil, organic sunflower seed oil, Udos
Choice Ultimate Oil Blend, walnut oil.

SOLGAR
Herts Tel: 01442 890355

Stocked by good independent health food shops.

● Nutrients: a large range of low to high dose vitamins,
minerals and antioxidant formulas.
● Essential fats: DHA, EPO, linseed oil, super EPA, super
GLA, wheat germ oil, one-a-day EPA/GLA.

ANTI-ALLERGY PRODUCTS

EXOREX
Tel: 01737 508 050

Management system (creams, shampoos, etc) for psoriasis (also
available on prescription).

GREEN PEOPLE
Tel: 01444 401 444

Website: www.greenpeople.co.uk
Natural cosmetics.

HEALTHY HOUSE
Tel: 01453 752 216
Allergy-free bedding and other supplies.

MARGARET EVANS
Tel: 01526 832 491
Mi-gon for migraine relief and SK eczema cream.

MEDIVAC
Tel: 01625 539 401
Specialised anti-allergy vacuum cleaners and other supplies.

PSORASOLV
Psoriasis ointment available from health shops

NUTRITIONAL THERAPISTS

BRITISH ASSOCIATION OF NUTRITIONAL THERAPISTS (BCM BANT)
London WC1N 3XX Tel: 0870 6061284

INSTITUTE FOR OPTIMUM NUTRITION (ION)
Blades Court, Deodar Road, London SW15 2NU. Tel: 020 8877 9993

BRITISH SOCIETY FOR ALLERGY, ENVIRONMENTAL AND NUTRITIONAL MEDICINE (BSAENM)
Southampton Tel: 01703 812 124.
Website: www.bsaenm.org.uk
For a list of medical doctors who have a particular interest in nutrition.

SOCIETY FOR THE PROMOTION OF NUTRITIONAL THERAPY

P.O. Box 626, Woking GU22 0XD. Tel: 01483 740 903
http://visitweb.com/spnt/

BIOCHEMICAL TESTING

GREAT SMOKIES DIAGNOSTIC LABORATORY

The services of this laboratory, which include adrenal stress
test, oxidative stress, EFA profile, can be organised
through their UK agents:
Diagnostic Services Ltd Tel: 0151 922 6200
Health Interlink Ltd Tel: 01664 810 011

THE INDIVIDUAL WELLBEING DIAGNOSTIC LABORATORY

London SW3 Tel: 020 7730 7010
The services they offer include adrenal stress index and allergy
tests; they also run a clinic in addition to their postal
service. All tests are supported by a nutrition consultation.

ORGANIC FOOD SOURCES

THE SOIL ASSOCIATION

86 Colston Street, Bristol BS1 5BB. Tel: 0117 929 0661
The Soil Association provides a list of organic suppliers in the
UK, as well as publications on organic issues. Telephone to
check the price of the catalogue.

SIMPLY ORGANIC

Tel: 0845 1000 444
Website: www.simplyorganic.net
National delivery of organic produce.

WATER DISTILLER SUPPLIERS

AQUAPURE DISTILLATION
Tel: 020 8892 9010

FRESHWATER FILTER COMPANY
Tel: 020 8558 7495

THE FRESHWATER COMPANY
Tel: 0345 023998
Delivery service of pre-distilled water to the south east of
England.

HIGHER NATURE
Tel: 01435 882880

WHOLISTIC RESEARCH COMPANY
Tel: 01954 781074

BOOKS

Dietary Fats and Fatty Acids in Human Healthcare Nigel
Plummer, BioMED Publications Ltd (Available from Biocare –
see supplement companies above)

Fats that Heal and Fats that Kill Udo Erasmus, Alive Books,
1996

Food Allergy and Intolerance Dr Jonathan Brostoff and Linda
Gamblin, Bloomsbury, 1998

Talking Dirty with the Queen of Clean Linda Cobb, Simon &
Schuster UK, 2001

The Stress Protection Plan Suzannah Olivier, Collins & Brown,
2000

What the Label Doesn't Tell You Sue Dibb, Thorsons, 1997

Recipe books

Allergy-free Cookbook Michelle Berriedale-Johnson, Thorsons, 1999

Cooking Without Barbara Cousins, Thorsons, 1998

Optimum Nutrition Cookbook Patrick Holford and Judith Ridgeway, Piatkus, 2000

OTHER

REGISTER OF HOMEOPATHS
Tel: 020 7566 7800

THE FEINGOLD ASSOCIATION WEBSITE
www.feingold.org
For information about E-numbers and other factors in allergy and hyperactivity.

BUTEYKO WORKSHOPS
0800 016 7879
A breathing system to aid asthmatics.

POCKET
BOOKS

NATURAL HORMONE BALANCE
YOU ARE WHAT YOU EAT
Suzannah Olivier

Women today are questioning the wisdom of
turning to artificial hormones and other chemical
preparations and techniques to alleviate their
female problems. A natural, nutritional approach
can help with PMS, infertility, mood swings,
irregular cycles, osteoporosis, endometriosis,
fibroids, ovarian cysts, breast cancer
and other problems.

Now all the nutritional advice you need is brought
together in **NATURAL HORMONE BALANCE**,
using simple, effective programmes that use
everyday foods and inexpensive diets.

Suzannah Olivier, a qualified nutritionist, has
written this major new health series fighting
common ailments the nutritional way.

ISBN 0 671 02954 1
Price £6.99

POCKET
BOOKS

BANISH BLOATING
YOU ARE WHAT YOU EAT
Suzannah Olivier

Many women, even if they are skinny, have a
problem with bloating and associated discomfort.

Now **BANISH BLOATING** looks at all the
possible causes – whether digestive, hormonal,
drug related or a sluggish detox process – and
pinpoints the best nutritional advice to combat this
condition. With easy-to-follow advice, and using
common, everyday foods and supplements, as
well as hit lists of food and food combinations to
avoid, here is the most healthy and holistic way to
eliminate the misery and discomfort of bloating.

Suzannah Olivier, a qualified nutritionist, has
written this major new health series fighting
common ailments the nutritional way.

ISBN 0 671 02953 3
Price £6.99

POCKET
B O O K S

MAXIMISING ENERGY
YOU ARE WHAT YOU EAT
Suzannah Olivier

We all want more energy.

MAXIMISING ENERGY shows how anyone, even
when juggling busy work and family lives, can
improve their available energy. Using tried and
trusted nutritional techniques, this book comes up
with a series of suggestions for maintaining a
steady stream of energy and good blood sugar
levels. It also highlights the foods and eating
habits that sap our bodies of energy.
MAXIMISING ENERGY will help eliminate
fatigue syndromes, listlessness and exhaustion on
a long-term basis.

Suzannah Olivier, a qualified nutritionist, has
written this major new health series fighting
common ailments the nutritional way.

ISBN 0 671 02955 X
Price £6.99

THE DETOX MANUAL
YOU ARE WHAT YOU EAT
Suzannah Olivier

Beat cellulite, headaches, skin rashes, tiredness, bad breath, non-arthritic joint aches and nausea by following **THE DETOX MANUAL**. Every day we are bombarded with toxins and there is only one practical option for dealing with this toxic overload. Adjusting our diet will improve the detoxification mechanisms that our bodies have. The increased sense of well being experienced by people after following the programmes outlined in **THE DETOX MANUAL** can be amazing.

THE DETOX MANUAL continues the major new health series fighting common ailments the nutritional way. Suzannah Olivier, a qualified nutritionist, has written a groundbreaking series, which tailors detailed programmes to individual, common problems.

ISBN 0 671 03782 X
Price £6.99

**POCKET
BOOKS**

EATING FOR A PERFECT PREGNANCY
YOU ARE WHAT YOU EAT
Suzannah Olivier

The pregnant mother's diet is of prime importance
to the developing baby. Find out which are the best
foods in **EATING FOR A PERFECT
PREGNANCY**, a must-have book for expecting
mothers. Covering pre-conception right through to
breast feeding, this book advises on the impact that
nutrition has on mother and child. Full of
fascinating facts and practical advice, read this
book for an energetic and symptom free
pregnancy.

EATING FOR A PERFECT PREGNANCY
continues the major new health series fighting
common ailments the nutritional way. Suzannah
Olivier, a qualified nutritionist, has written a
groundbreaking series, which tailors detailed
programmes to individual, common problems.

ISBN 0 671 03781 1
Price £6.99

POCKET
B O O K S

This book and other health and nutrition titles are available from your bookshop or can be ordered direct from the publisher.

0 671 02954 1 **Natural Hormone Balance/Suzannah Olivier**   £6.99
0 671 02953 3 **Banish Bloating/Suzannah Olivier**   £6.99
0 671 02955 X **Maximising Energy/Suzannah Olivier**   £6.99
0 671 03781 1 **Eating for a Perfect Pregnancy /Suzannah Olivier** £6.99
0 671 03782 X **The Detox Manual/Suzannah Olivier**   £6.99
0 671 77377 1 **Potatoes Not Prozac/Kathleen DesMaisons**   £6.99
0 671 03735 8 **Food Your Miracle Medicine/Jean Carper**   £8.99
0 671 03736 6 **The Food Pharmacy/Jean Carper**   £8.99

Please send cheque or postal order for the value of the book, free postage and packing within the UK; OVERSEAS including Republic of Ireland £1 per book.

OR: Please debit this amount from my

VISA/ACCESS/MASTERCARD ....

CARD NO: ....

EXPIRY DATE ....

AMOUNT£ ....

NAME ....

ADDRESS ....

....

SIGNATURE ....

Send orders to SIMON & SCHUSTER CASH SALES
PO Box 29, Douglas Isle of Man, IM99 1BQ
Tel: 01624 836000, Fax: 01624 670923
www.bookpost.co.uk
Please allow 14 days for delivery. Prices and availability
subject to change without notice